Key Developments
in
Gastroenterology

Key Developments
in
Gastroenterology

Edited by

P. R. SALMON
The Middlesex Hospital, London

A Wiley Medical Publication

JOHN WILEY & SONS
Chichester · New York · Brisbane · Toronto · Singapore

British Library Cataloguing in Publication Data

Salmon, P.R. (Paul Raymond)
  Key developments in gastroenterology.
  1. Medicine.   Gastroenterology
  I. Title
  616.3'3

  ISBN 0 471 91584 X

Typeset by Witwell Ltd, Southport.
Printed and bound in Great Britain by Bath Press Ltd, Bath

Contributors

D.G. Colin-Jones, *Queen Alexandra Hospital, Portsmouth, Hampshire*

D.P. Jewell, *Radcliffe Infirmary and University of Oxford, Oxford*

M.J.S. Langman, *Queen Elizabeth Hospital, Birmingham*

W.R. Lees, *The Middlesex Hospital, London*

J.J. Misiewicz, *The Middlesex Hospital, London*

R.J. Polson, *King's College Hospital and School of Medicine and Dentistry, London*

R.E. Pounder, *Royal Free Hospital School of Medicine, London*

W.D.W. Rees, *Hope Hospital, University of Manchester School of Medicine, Salford, Manchester*

S. Sherlock, *Royal Free Hospital School of Medicine, London*

C.J. Shorrock, *Hope Hospital, University of Manchester School of Medicine, Salford, Manchester*

P.M. Smith, *Llandough Hospital, Cardiff*

H.C. Thomas, *St Mary's Hospital and Medical School, University of London, London*

I.V.D. Weller, *University College and Middlesex Hospital Medical School, London*

R. Williams, *King's College Hospital and School of Medicine and Dentistry, London*

R.C.N. Williamson, *Bristol Royal Infirmary, Bristol*

Contents

Acknowledgement

This publication is based upon presentations given at 'The Glaxo Symposium 1986' held in Edinburgh 10–12 December 1986 by Glaxo Laboratories Ltd.

Key Developments in Gastroenterology
Edited by P. R. Salmon
© 1988 John Wiley & Sons Ltd

1

Modern Management
of Chronic Viral Hepatitis

Howard C. Thomas
St Mary's Hospital and Medical School, University of London, London

Chronic HBV Infection

Factors influencing response

Patients with this condition are heterogeneous in terms of:

1) Time of infection (neonatal in Japanese and Chinese; early childhood in Africa; early adult life in Western Europe and North America)
2) Duration of infection
3) Severity of hepatitis
4) Immune status (homosexual patients have a second-degree immuno-deficiency unrelated to HIV (Regenstein et al, 1983) infection and also, in some cases, to HIV infection).

Neonatal infection, long duration of infection, immunodeficiency and low inflammatory activity may reduce probability of response (Scullard et al, 1981c).

Indications for therapy (not definitely identified)

1) Infectivity—HBe antigen and HBV-DNA positive patients
2) Evidence of progressive liver disease—histological evidence of chronic active hepatitis.

Contra-indication for therapy

Evidence of decompensated cirrhosis

Goals of therapy

1) Inhibition of HBV replication (by direct effect or by stimulation of the host antiviral response)
2) Long-term control of inflammatory necrosis of hepatocytes
3) Prevention of malignant transformation of hepatocytes.

Responses may be of three types (Figures 1 and 2)

1) Transient response

Transient inhibition of HBV replication—loss of HBV-DNA and DNA polymerase but not HBeAg or HBsAg during therapy *but* return of these markers on cessation of therapy.

2) Incomplete response

Sustained inhibition of HBV replication—loss of HBV-DNA and DNA polymerase continuing after cessation of therapy, conversion from HBeAg to anti-HBe *but* continued HBs antigenaemia (due to translation of integrated HBV-DNA).

3) Complete response

Sustained inhibition of HBV replication—loss of HBV-DNA and DNA polymerase continuing after cessation of therapy, with permanent sero-conversion from HBsAg and HBeAg to anti-HBs and anti-HBe.

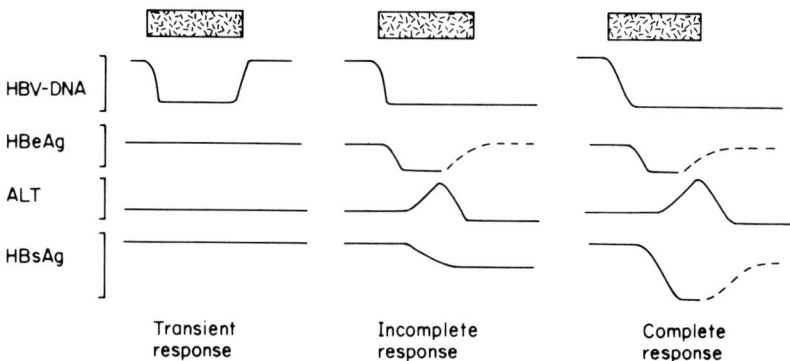

Figure 1. Pattern of response to antiviral treatment.

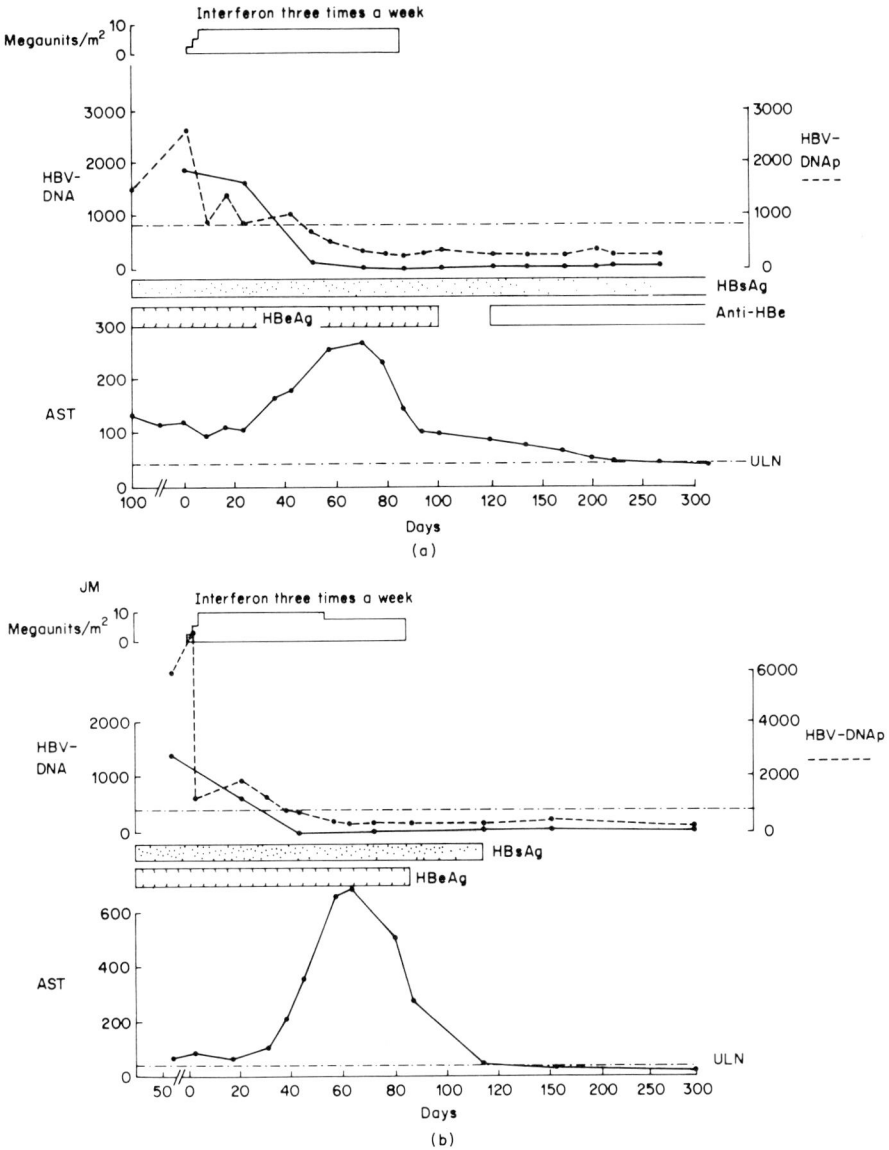

Figure 2. (a) *Incomplete response:* Inhibition of HBV replication associated with a transient exacerbation and then normalisation of the liver function tests. Note the patient remains HBsAg positive, presumably because of the presence of integrated HBV sequences. Benefits to the patient include reduced infectivity and cessation of inflammatory liver disease. (b) *Complete response:* inhibition of HBV replication and clearance of HBs antigen.

Active drugs: summary of controlled trial data

1) *Adenine arabinoside*

Potent inhibitor of HBV replication but clinical usefulness limited by poor aqueous solubility. In one small, randomised, controlled study a 10-day course produced sustained or temporary HBe antigen/antibody seroconversion in 40% of cases (Bassendine et al, 1981).

2) *Adenine arabinoside monophosphate*

Equally effective inhibitor of HBV replication which can be given by IM bolus injection twice daily (Scullard et al, 1981; Weller et al, 1982). A course of 10 mg/kg/24 h for three days followed by 5 mg/kg/24 h for a further 23 days has been evaluated in three controlled studies (Hoofnagle et al, 1984; Trepo et al, 1984; Weller et al, 1985) (Table 1).

Table 1

Author	HBeAg to anti-HBe conversion (1 year)		P values	Comment
	Control	ARA-MP		
Hoofnagle *et al.*	1/10	4/10	NS	Reactivation by 18–24 months
Weller *et al.*	0/14	6/15	$P < 0.05$	Complicated by intercurrent HAV and HDV
Trepo *et al.*	5/19	10/19	$P < 0.05$	Repeat courses given
TOTAL	6/43	20/44		

Conclusion: ARA-AMP at least triples HBeAg/anti-HBe seroconversion rate, but still less than half of patients respond.

Variability of response may be related to heterogeneity of patient populations being studied (see earlier). In one study none of 24 homosexual HBV carriers responded whereas 10/22 heterosexual (predominantly southern European) carriers did (Thomas et al, 1987) (Figure 3).

3) *Acycloguanosine (acyclovir)*

Active in low concentrations in herpes simplex because of phosphorylation to active metabolites by virus encoded thymidine kinase. This enzyme is not present in HBV-infected cells so this mode of action does not operate. Higher concentrations (near the maximum tolerated) give approximately 25% inhibition of HBV replication (Sidwell et al, 1982; Weller et al, 1983) but this has not been shown to be clinically useful.

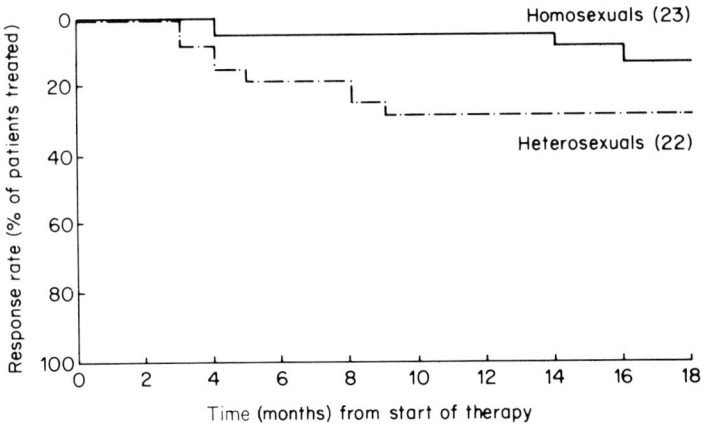

Figure 3. Response (= loss of HBeAg) to ARA-AMP (28 days, twice a week) in homosexual and heterosexual men. (Weller et al, 1984; Lok et al, 1986).

4) *Type I interferon (alpha and beta)*

Both natural and recombinant DNA produced preparations have been examined.

a) *Leucocyte alpha IFN* has been shown to inhibit HBV replication when given daily in moderate doses (5–10 megaunits/m^2/day over three to six months) (Greenberg et al, 1976). A randomised controlled study showed that low doses for four to six weeks produced no long-term responses (Schalm and Heijtink, 1982). Longer courses of moderate doses have not been evaluated in controlled studies.

b) *Lymphoblastoid alpha IFN*, given three times a week for three months in moderate doses, has been compared with ARA-MP (Los et al, 1983). Forty five per cent of patients showed long-term inhibition of HBV replication. Although no control group was included in this study, this response rate is nine times the average annual spontaneous seroconversion rate seen in the same population of patients (Viola et al, 1981). Further analysis of this study showed that Chinese carriers (presumably infected from birth) showed no response whereas European carriers exhibited a 55% conversion rate (Thomas and Scully, 1985) (Figures 4 and 5).

c) *Recombinant alpha IFN*, given daily in high doses, inhibits HBV replication but is toxic (Smith et al, 1983). Moderate doses (10 megaunits/m^2 daily or three times a week) are better tolerated and can be given for three to six months (McDonald et al, 1986). Several large randomised controlled studies are in progress.

d) *Beta IFNs* of natural and recombinant types have been used and shown to have similar activity to alpha IFN. No controlled studies are reported.

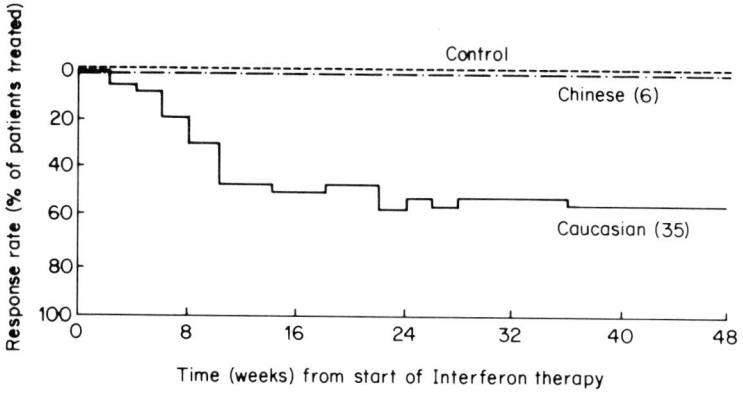

Figure 4. Response (= loss of HBeAg) to alpha interferon (3–6 months, three times a week) in Chinese and Caucasian HBV carriers (Scully et al, 1986).

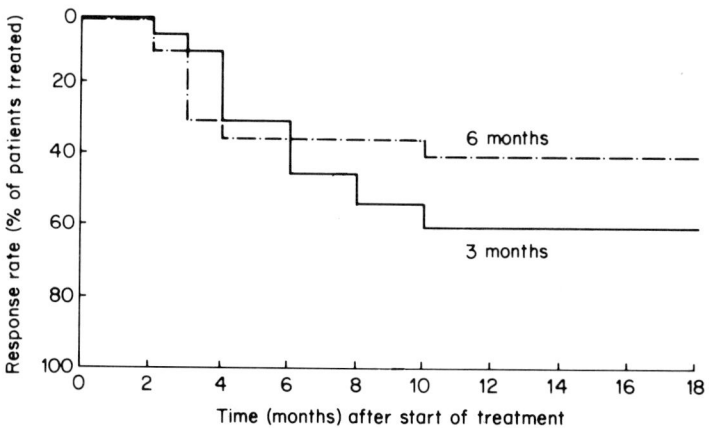

Figure 5. Response (= loss of HBeAg) to lymphoblastoid interferon: comparison of three and six months' therapy (Scully et al, 1986).

5) Type II interferon (gamma)

Both natural and recombinant are available. These are predominantly immunostimulant with less direct antiviral activity. Inhibition of HBV replication does occur after several months therapy. The optimal dosaging is not established.

6) *Interleukin II*

This is a lymphokine which amplifies immune function. It has been tried safely in individual patients but its place has not been established.

7) *Combination therapy*

a) *Short course prednisolone plus antiviral therapy (ARA-MP or IFN)*: Withdrawal of immunosuppressant therapy may result in HBeAg/Ab seroconversion (Scullard et al, 1981; Weller et al, 1982). However, short courses of prednisolone (one or two months) do not, on cessation, precipitate seroconversion (Hoofnagle et al, 1986). When followed by ARA-MP or alpha IFN, 60–70% seroconversion rates have been reported in small controlled studies (Perrillo et al, 1985). This requires further study. Care must be taken when withdrawing steroids particularly in patients with severe liver disease—fatalities have been recorded.

b) *Acyclovir and alpha interferon:* Preliminary studies suggest that there may be an advantage in this approach (Schalm et al, 1985).

General comments

Inhibition of viral replication, associated with HBe antigen/antibody seroconversion, is usually long-lasting and accompanied, after a transient exacerbation, by amelioration of the inflammatory liver disease (Figure 2). Reactivation may occur, particularly in homosexual patients with or without HIV infection (Davis and Hoofnagle, 1985).

If integration of HBV sequences into the host cell genome has occurred before starting treatment, HBs antigenaemia will continue after cessation of detectable HBV replication (Figure 2b). However, inflammatory liver disease will ameliorate in these patients if long-term inhibition of HBV replication is achieved.

Patients treated early in the course of the disease will lose HBs antigen from their serum if cessation of HBV replication is achieved (Figure 2a).

Chronic Delta Virus Infection

Preliminary data indicate that levels of HDV-RNA in serum are reduced by administration of alpha interferons (Hoofnagle, pers. comm.; Farci et al, 1987) but the effects on the course of the disease have not been studied.

Chronic Non-A, Non-B Virus Infection

The failure of investigators to identify serological systems for the diagnosis of non-A, non-B infection and of methods to measure viral replication has impeded the development of adequate therapy. Antiviral drugs would be a logical approach but have not been tried.

References

Bassendine MF, Chadwick RG, Salmeron J et al (1981) Adenine arabinoside therapy in HBsAg-positive chronic liver disease: a controlled study. *Gastroenterology* **80**, 1016–22.

Davis GL and Hoofnagle JH (1985) Reactivation of chronic type B hepatitis presenting as acute viral hepatitis. *Ann. Int. Med.* **102**, 762–5.

Farci P, Shuir R, Karayiannis P et al (1987) Inhibition of delta virus replication by lymphoblastoid human alpha interferon. *Gut* (in press).

Greenberg HB, Pollard RB, Lutwick LI et al (1976) Effect of human leukocyte interferon on hepatitis B virus infection in patients with chronic active hepatitis. *New Engl. J. Med.* **295**, 517–22.

Hoofnagle JH, Hansor RG, Minuk GY et al (1984) Randomized controlled trial of adenine arabinoside monophosphate for chronic type B hepatitis. *Gastroenterology* **86**, 150–7.

Hoofnagle JH, Davis GL, Pappas SC et al (1986) A short course of prednisolone in chronic type B hepatitis. *Ann. Int. Med.* **104**, 12–17.

Hoofnagle J. Personal communication.

Lok ASF, Karayiannis P, Brown D et al (1983) A randomised study of the effect of adenine arabinoside monophosphate (4 or 8 week courses) versus lymphoblastoid interferon on hepatitis B virus (HBV) replication. *Hepatology* **3**, 865 (abstract 268).

McDonald J, Caruso L and Thomas HC (1986) A randomised controlled trial of recombinant alpha interferon in treatment of HBV infection. *Hepatology* (AASLD meeting abstract).

Perrillo RP, Regerstein FG, Bodicky CJ et al (1985) Comparative efficacy of ARA-MP in prednisolone withdrawal followed by ARA-MP in treatment of HBV induced CAH. *Gastroenterology* **88**, 780–6.

Regenstein FG, Roodman ST and Perillo RP (1983) Immunoregulatory T cells subsets in chronic hepatitis B virus infection: the influence of homosexuality. *Hepatology* **3**, 951–4.

Schalm SW and Heijtink RA (1982) Spontaneous disappearance of viral replication and liver cell inflammation in HBs-Ag positive chronic active hepatitis: results of a placebo vs. interferon trial. *Hepatology* **2**, 791–4.

Schalm SW, Heytick RA, van Buuren HR and de Man RA (1985) Acyclovir enhances the antiviral effect of interferon in chronic hepatitis B. *Lancet* **17**, 358–60.

Scullard GH, Andres LL, Greenberg HB et al (1981a) Antiviral treatment of chronic hepatitis B virus infection: improvement in liver disease with interferon and adenine arabinoside. *Hepatology* **1**, 228–32.

Scullard GGH, Smith IC, Merigan TC, Robinson WS and Gregory PB (1981b) Effects of immunosuppressive therapy on viral markers in chronic active hepatitis B. *Gastroenterology* **81**, 987–91.

Scullard GH, Pollard RB, Smith JL et al (1981c) Antiviral treatment of chronic hepatitis B virus infection: changes in viral markers with interferon combined with adenine arabinoside. *J. Infect. Dis.* **143**, 772–83.

Sidwell RW, Huffman JH, Khare GP et al (1982) Broad-spectrum antiviral activity of virazole: I-ß-D ribofuranosyl-1,2,4-triazole 3-carboxamide. *Science* **177**, 705–6.

Smith CI, Weissberg J, Bernhardt L et al (1983) Acute Dane particle suppression with leukocyte recombinant interferon in chronic HBV infection. *J. Infect. Dis.* **148**, 907–13.

Thomas HC and Scully LJ (1985) Antiviral therapy in hepatitis B infection. *Brit. Med. Bull.* **41**, 374–80.

Thomas HC, Lever AML, Scully LJ and Pignatelli M (1987) Approaches to the treatment of HBV and HDV related liver disease. *Seminars in Liver Disease* **6**, 34–41.

Trepo C, Hantz O, Ouzan D et al (1984) Therapeutic efficacy of ARA-MP in symptomatic HBe Ag positive C A H: a randomized, placebo control study. *Hepatology* **4**, 1055 (abstract 193).

Viola LA, Barrison IG and Coleman JC et al (1981) Natural history of liver disease in chronic hepatitis B surface antigen carriers. Survey of 100 patients from Great Britain. *Lancet* **2**, 1156–9.

Weller IVD, Bassendine MF, Craxi et al (1982) Successful treatment of HBs and HBeAg positive chronic liver disease: prolonged inhibition of viral replication by highly soluble adenine arabinoside 5'-monophosphate (ARA-MP). *Gut* **23**, 717–23.

Weller IVD, Bassendine MF, Murray AK et al (1982) Effects of prednisolone/azathioprine in chronic B viral hepatitis. *Gut* **23**, 650–5.

Weller IVD, Carreno V, Fowler MJF et al (1983) Acyclovir in hepatitis B antigen-positive chronic liver disease: inhibition of viral replication and transient renal impairment with iv bolus administration. *J. Antimicrob. Chemother.* **11**, 223–31.

Weller IVD, Lok ASF, Mindel A et al (1985) A randomised controlled trial of adenine arabinoside 5'-monophosphate (ARA-MP) in chronic hepatitis B virus infection. *Gut* **26**, 745–51.

Key Developments in Gastroenterology
Edited by P. R. Salmon
© 1988 John Wiley & Sons Ltd

2

The Modern Management of Bleeding Oesophageal Varices

P.M. Smith

Llandough Hospital, Cardiff

Introduction

Bleeding from oesophageal varices can be terrifying for the patient, with an initial mortality of at least 25%. Portal hypertension is usually secondary to cirrhosis, but extrahepatic portal vein block and non-cirrhotic portal fibrosis can also be responsible; the commonest cause in the world is schistosomiasis.

For varices to develop, portal hypertension must be present but the risk of bleeding depends principally on variceal size (Lebrec et al, 1980a). As the varix distends, its wall becomes thinner and wall stress increases.

Resuscitation

The first priority in management is resuscitation. Blood transfusion is required. Attempts to correct platelet counts and clotting factors are of little value in an emergency since their half-life is short and they are unlikely to affect variceal bleeding. Intravenous saline must be avoided as it will induce ascites and oedema. The physical signs of cirrhosis should be looked for and a history of alcoholism or previous liver disease sought.

Diagnosis

Upper gastrointestinal endoscopy should be performed as soon as possible. Even though varices have been demonstrated previously by radiology, peptic ulcers are common in cirrhotics, and haemorrhagic gastritis can occur in alcoholics; these non-variceal sources must be excluded.

Treatment of the Acute Bleed

If bleeding has ceased at the time of endoscopy, and the patient is no longer shocked, sclerotherapy should be performed. If the patient is bleeding actively, however, this will be difficult, and the haemorrhage must be stopped. Blood transfusion will be wasted if blood loss continues at a rapid rate.

Balloon tamponade

This can be most effective, bleeding ceasing in 86% (Teres et al, 1978) and 87% (Sarin and Nundy, 1984). Provided the gastric balloon is well within the stomach before inflation, there should be few complications. However, pressure necrosis of the oesophageal wall can occur if the oesophageal balloon is left inflated for more than 24 hours. Aspiration pneumonia is less common with the four-lumen Minnesota tube than with the three-lumen Sengstaken tube, the extra lumen allowing pharyngeal suction.

Tamponade should be regarded as a temporary measure, allowing resuscitation and control of haemorrhage prior to sclerotherapy or transection. The patient is then taken to theatre and the balloon removed only at the time of treatment.

Vasopressin therapy

Vasopressin infusion has been used to treat bleeding oesophageal varices for 30 years. It causes constriction of mesenteric arterioles, thus reducing the inflow of blood to the portal venous system and the varices. This was almost as effective as balloon tamponade in one trial (Pinto Correia et al, 1984). A critical review, however, concluded that continuous intravenous infusion of 0.5–0.6 units/min produces temporary arrest of variceal bleeding in 50–70% (placebo 0–30%), without any effect on the ultimate survival rate (Hussey, 1985). In a controlled trial, 93% of patients treated with oesophageal tamponade as well as vasopressin stopped bleeding, but this was not significantly different from the 78% of control patients treated by tamponade only (Clanet et al, 1978). These results and those from another trial (Merigan et al, 1962) suggest that there is no advantage in treatment with vasopressin once oesophageal tamponade has been established. Vasopressin also has a number of vasoconstrictor side-effects, including systemic hypertension, abdominal pain and coronary vasoconstriction. The simultaneous administration of nitroglycerin (40–400 μg/min) will reverse the vasoconstrictor side-effects on the systemic arteriolar system, without affecting the diminution of portal pressure and portal inflow (Gimson et al, 1986). Although this does not lessen transfusion requirements or improve survival, it allows larger doses of vasopressin to be given without side-effects.

Glypressin

Triglycyl lysine vasopressin is a vasopressin analogue. It has very little activity on smooth muscle, but cleavage of terminal amino acid residues results in the slow release of active hormone, smooth muscle constriction being maintained for up to 10 hours by a single injection, whereas an equipotent dose of vasopressin is active for only 20–40 minutes. Freeman et al (1982) showed that glypressin (2 mg six-hourly) controlled bleeding in 70% of cirrhotic patients with bleeding varices, as compared to only 9% who received a constant infusion of vasopressin (0.4 units/min). The glypressin group required significantly less blood and had no side-effects. However, Silk et al (1979) controlled bleeding in only 33% of patients with glypressin.

Somatostatin

Somatostatin, first discovered in 1973, occurs in the brain, the pancreas and the gastric antrum, and in lower concentrations in the small and large intestine and the thyroid. It inhibits the secretion of growth hormone and thyroid-stimulating hormone by the pituitary, insulin and glucagon by the pancreas, and various gastrointestinal hormones by the gut. It is a powerful inhibitor of gastric acid secretion. In addition, it acts directly on mesenteric vascular smooth muscle, reducing portal pressure. Jenkins et al (1985) compared vasopressin with somatostatin and concluded that the latter was much more effective and without complications. In two uncontrolled studies, intravenous infusion of somatostatin stopped bleeding from oesophageal varices in all cirrhotic patients treated (Thulin et al, 1979; Tyden et al, 1978). However, in other studies somatostatin had no effect on bleeding varices (Raptis and Zoupas, 1979) or on hepatic blood flow and wedged hepatic vein pressure (Sonnenburg et al, 1981). Furthermore, somatostatin is very expensive. Its routine use therefore depends upon results from further controlled trials.

Vasoconstrictor drugs offer only temporary control when effective. Thirty per cent of patients will rebleed within a week without further treatment and 75% will rebleed within six months.

Long-Term Treatment of Bleeding Varices

Pharmacological treatment

Lebrec et al (1980b) reported that propranolol would reduce the wedged hepatic venous pressure by decreasing cardiac output and, secondarily, splanchnic and hepatic blood flow. A controlled study of propranolol in patients with oesophageal varices and cirrhosis followed. Of 38 patients treated with propranolol in a dose sufficient to reduce the heart rate by 25%, only one bled over a one-year period. In contrast, 18 out of 36 patients treated by a placebo rebled during the same period. During the second year only 21% bled in the propranolol group as opposed to 68% in the control group. Survival also improved with treatment (Lebrec et al, 1984; Figure 1). The majority of patients, however,

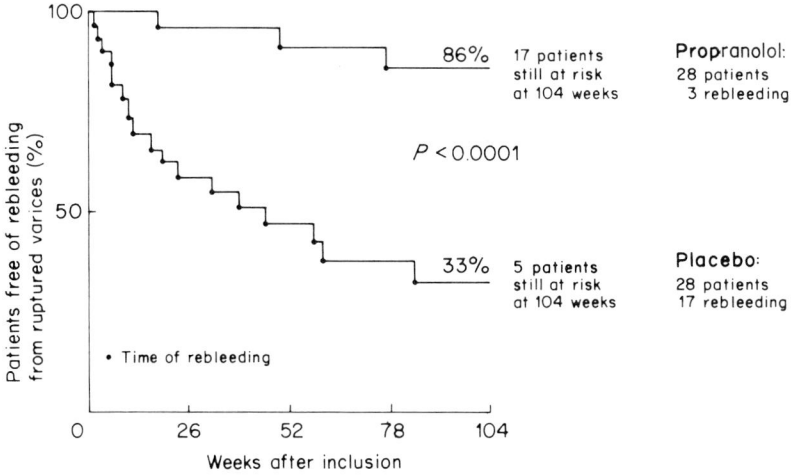

Figure 1. Percentages of patients free of rebleeding as a function of time after inclusion among the subjects who bled from ruptured varices in the propranolol and the placebo group. (The percentages were calculated by the Kaplan-Meier method and compared by the log rank test.) From Lebrec et al (1984), *Hepatology* **4**, 355–8, by kind permission of the editor of the journal and the author. © American Association for the Study of Liver Disease.

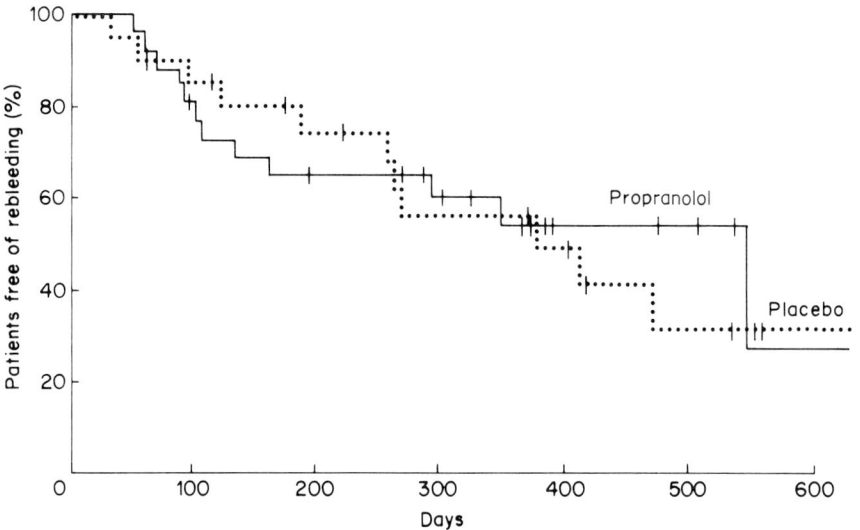

Figure 2. Percentages of patients who had bled from varices without rebleeding after inclusion in the study in propranolol and placebo groups. By kind permission of the Editor of the *New England Journal of Medicine*.

had compensated cirrhosis and 25% bled from gastric erosions rather than varices.

Lebrec et al (1980a) have also stated that there is no relationship between the risk of haemorrhage from varices and the portal venous pressure, so it is surprising that propranolol works. A trial in London, however, found no decrease in the bleeding incidence in the propranolol-treated group over two years' follow-up (Burroughs et al, 1983; Figure 2), in spite of a significant reduction in wedged hepatic vein pressure. Furthermore, several side-effects follow propranolol administration to cirrhotics. They include a rise in arterial ammonia levels, a decline in the ability to perform a number connection test, a worsening of encephalopathy and inability of the circulation to respond adequately to haemorrhage (Conn, 1984).

Propranolol may be more effective at reducing portal pressure than a selective $ß_1$-receptor blocker. The additional effect of propranolol may be due to the $ß_2$-receptor blockade of splanchnic vessels, leading to unopposed vasoconstriction and a reduction in splanchnic blood flow. Oral metoprolol, a selective $ß$-blocker, was given to 15 patients with oesophageal varices in a controlled trial (Westaby et al, 1985a). Nine (60%) rebled during an 18-month follow-up, three times as many as in the comparable group treated with sclerotherapy.

In summary, propranolol may reduce the portal pressure, but it is not yet proven that it can reduce the incidence of variceal bleeding in cirrhosis, and it has some unwelcome side effects.

Transhepatic injection of varices

Lunderquist and Vang (1974) devised a percutaneous transhepatic approach to the portal system, with catheterisation and embolisation of the left gastric and coronary veins supplying the oesophageal varices. The technique requires considerable radiological skill, taking 2–4 hours. Catheters may be difficult to manipulate in a small cirrhotic liver, and anatomical variations cause difficulties.

The technique is successful in 73–87% of cases, but rebleeding occurs in 40–65% (Dick, 1981). Although recanalisation of blocked varices occurs, the major problem is the formation of new collaterals. Complications include bleeding from the liver, biliary peritonitis and portal vein thrombosis, which can occur in 25–40% of cases.

Because of these problems, transhepatic injection has now been largely replaced by injection sclerotherapy (see below).

Laser therapy

This is still in its infancy. Haemostasis was achieved in 92% of bleeding varices in one series, but the rebleeding rate was 30% (Kiefhaber et al, 1983). Fleischer (1985) compared 10 patients with varices treated by Nd:YAG laser with 10 controls. Initial haemostasis was achieved in seven laser-treated patients but in 0 out of the 10 controls receiving sham treatment. However four of the seven initially controlled with laser therapy rebled 12–48 hours later. The laser was aimed around the bleeding point, but caused acute haemorrhage in two patients. Treatment did not affect blood transfusion requirements. Fleischer concluded that laser therapy was not definitive but could be used as an interim solution.

Surgery

Portacaval shunting will reduce portal pressure to normal, effectively preventing variceal bleeding, but the procedure has a number of important drawbacks. The operative mortality may be high, hepatic failure and encephalopathy may follow diversion of the portal blood away from the liver, and in some cases encephalopathy appears only after the shunt, the risk increasing with time. From 1945, however, the portacaval shunt was the usual method employed to deal with variceal bleeding. In 1968 Conn and Lindenmuth demonstrated that prophylactic shunting of cirrhotic patients with varices led to a slight increase in mortality as compared with a control group, hepatic failure replacing variceal haemorrhage as the principal cause of death. This was followed by two other trials (Rueff et al, 1976; Resnick et al, 1974) which demonstrated that the therapeutic shunt did not prolong life and induced encephalopathy in a significant number of patients. Rueff et al concluded that portacaval shunting could no longer be accepted as a suitable treatment for cirrhotic patients with gastrointestinal bleeding.

Various modifications of the standard end-to-side portacaval shunt were therefore introduced, including side-to-side, double-barrelled, mesocaval and splenorenal shunts, but all had similar side-effects. Since total hepatic blood flow is reduced by 40–50% after a shunt (Price et al, 1967), attempts have been made to arterialise the portal vein using the splenic artery (Maillard et al, 1974) or a vein graft from the right common iliac artery. The results of a long-term follow-up are still awaited.

In 1967 Warren et al described the distal splenorenal shunt with portal azygous disconnection in an attempt to selectively decompress the portal systemic collateral veins around the stomach and oesophagus, while preserving portal venous blood flow. The original report suggested that variceal bleeding was well-controlled and encephalopathy and hepatic failure were less common (Warren et al, 1974), although the operation was difficult and there was an increased operative mortality. Six prospective randomised clinical trials have compared the distal splenorenal shunt with the standard portacaval shunt, and all have found that survival was not improved. Three studies showed a significantly lower encephalopathy rate for the selective shunt but the other three did not. One trial (Harley et al, 1986) demonstrated a significantly higher variceal rebleeding rate. Warren and his colleagues (1986) have recently demonstrated in a preliminary report that endoscopic sclerotherapy, despite a high rebleeding rate, gives better liver function and improved survival when compared with the distal splenorenal shunt, and a report from Barcelona (Teres et al, 1986) found the mortality, survival and days of hospitalisation were similar for the two procedures, although the distal shunt had a higher encephalopathy rate.

Oesophageal transection

Walker (1964) realised that varices tend to bleed at the level of the oesophago-gastric junction, and that stopping venous flow at this level by transection was effective via a thoracotomy incision. The procedure was simplified by the advent of the stapling gun and the use of an abdominal incision. Combining transection with devascularisation of the lower oesophagus, Johnston (1982) treated 80 patients with bleeding varices with a hospital mortality rate of only 14% and a three-year survival rate of 69%. Encephalopathy was not a problem, although late recurrent bleeding occurred in 14 patients. When oesophageal transaction was compared with a mesocaval shunt, transection was found to have a lower operative mortality and a lower incidence of encephalopathy, yet with an equal rebleeding rate (Osborne and Hobbs, 1981), although the rebleeding rate increased with time (Hamilton et al, 1984).

   In Japan, Sugiura performed para-oesophagogastric devascularisation with oesophageal transection, with a low mortality and a very low incidence of recurrent variceal bleeding (Sugiura and Futagawa, 1984). His results have not been reproduced in Europe, however, perhaps because only 16% of Sugiura's patients required an emergency procedure, 30% merely undergoing a prophylactic one. Furthermore, only 73% had cirrhosis, and in the great majority this was non-alcoholic.

Injection sclerotherapy

Injection sclerotherapy for oesophageal varices was first described in 1939, but lapsed because of the introduction of portacaval shunting which became the accepted treatment. When controlled trials showed no advantage for shunting over simple medical treatment in the 1970s, interest in sclerotherapy revived and, aided by the introduction of the fibrescope, led to re-evaluation of the technique; over 500 papers have been published in the last five years.

   Variceal haemorrhage occurs through a pinhole in the vein wall, rather than by erosion. It is intermittent, and may stop spontaneously. Bleeding occurs within 2 cm of the gastro-oesophageal junction. Blood loss above this level is rare but up to 5% of patients may bleed from gastric varices in the fundus. Varices receive blood from the left gastric vein, a branch of the portal vein, and the short gastric veins that arise from branches of the splenic vein. Both sets of veins run in the submucosa of the stomach, and 2–3 cm below the gastro-oesophageal junction are grouped longitudinally together as gastric varices (De Carvalho, 1966). At the gastro-oesophageal junction, parallel longitudinal veins cross the muscularis mucosa to lie superficially in the lamina propria. The vessels pass back into the submucosa 2–3 cm further up (Noda, 1984), from where they continue an upward course as four or five large vessels until they penetrate the muscular wall of the oesophagus to join the azygous system.

McCormack et al (1983) studied blood flow patterns in the oesophageal varices by Doppler ultrasonography and injection radiography. They showed that blood flow at the lower end of the gullet may be either towards the head or towards the stomach, the direction varying with respiration. They concluded that there were perforating veins joining the varices to perioesophageal veins; these perforators have been demonstrated anatomically by resin casts (Kitano et al, 1986). The development of incompetent perforating veins may be analogous to the situation in the leg when varicose veins arise. As in the leg, successful sclerotherapy depends on destroying the incompetent perforating veins and the main variceal channels.

These findings offer an anatomical explanation for the fact that variceal bleeding is limited to within 2–3 cm of the gastro-oesophageal junction, and show why sclerotherapy should be limited to this area alone. Bleeding from gastric varices occurs in only 5% of patients, and is associated with very large clusters of vessels. Retrograde thrombosis of gastric varices can actually follow intravariceal injection within the oesophagus, the sclerosant being carried into the gastric varices by downward flow (McCormack et al, 1983). There is a high incidence of early rebleeding, however, and the survival rate is lower than that for oesophageal bleeders (Trudeau and Prindiville, 1986; Figure 3).

Technique

Originally, rigid endoscopy was performed under general anaesthesia. Nowadays diazemuls analgesia, with intravenous buscopan to paralyse the oesophagus, allows the passage of a fibrescope, which is safe and simple to use. An end viewing instrument with a bridge to alter the angle of the injecting needle, or an oblique viewing endoscope are preferable. An instrument with a widebore biopsy channel provides better suction facilities if haemorrhage occurs.

The flexible oesophageal sheath developed at King's College Hospital, London, has a distal slot into which the varix prolapses, allowing easy injection. Other groups have used a compressing balloon either above or below the site of injection in order to provide a bloodless field. No convincing evidence to show an advantage for these techniques has yet been presented, and many endoscopists believe that these devices complicate sclerotherapy without providing any benefits.

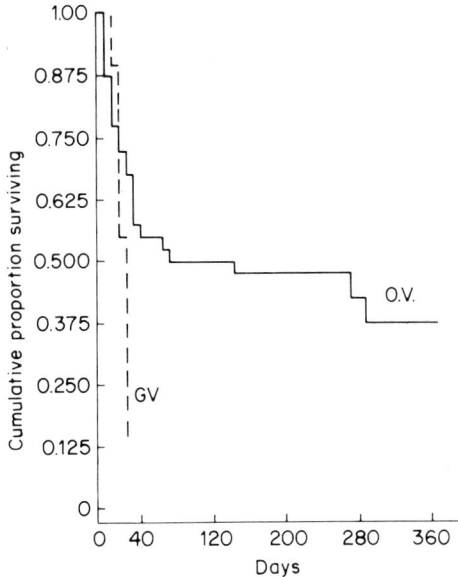

Figure 3. Survival of patients with gastric varices (GV) and oesophageal varices (OV). Kaplan-Meier analysis. From Trudeau and Prindiville (1986), *Gastrointestinal Endoscopy* **32**, 264–8, by kind permission of the editor of the journal and the author. © American Society for Gastrointestinal Endoscopy.

If the patient is actively bleeding at the time of endoscopy, accurate intravariceal injection is very difficult, although the rigid endoscope has been used to control active bleeding by pressure on the cardia (Spence et al, 1985). Most endoscopists control haemorrhage with a Sengstaken-Blakemore tube, removing the tube at a convenient time within the next 2–24 hours in the endoscopy theatre immediately prior to treatment. If recurrent bleeding is life threatening or it renders further sclerotherapy impracticable, oesophageal transection with a stapling gun provides a period of 3–12 months during which follow-up sclerotherapy can be used to deal with any variceal recurrence.

At endoscopy it is important to document the position and size of the varices at the lower end of the oesophagus, using a clock face system and grading the varices subjectively on a scale of 1–4. Using this system of record keeping, it is possible to follow the steady reduction in size and eventual disappearance of the varices.

The sclerosant is injected via a fine-bore long needle passed down the biopsy channel of the instrument. Up to 2 ml of sclerosant is injected into each varix just above the gastro-oesophageal junction. Bleeding is only occasionally precipitated, and can be dealt with by the passage of a Sengstaken tube for 1 hour. Further injections are performed weekly until the varices have shrunk, when the risk of bleeding is reduced (Rose et al, 1983). Thereafter, monthly injections, on a day admission basis, continue until all varices are thrombosed. Between 1 and 13 injections are required to complete treatment, but the larger the varix the more injections required (Rose et al, 1983).

Crafoord and Frenckner (1939) used quinine as a sclerosant in the first reported case of injection sclerotherapy. Subsequently, sodium morrhuate was used (Macbeth, 1955). Blenkinsopp (1968), using the rat femoral vein, demonstrated that sodium tetradecyl sulphate (STD) was superior to ethanolamine oleate as a thrombotic agent, both agents producing similar degrees of tissue necrosis when injected subcutaneously. Ethanolamine is more viscous than STD, and is more likely to cause 'sclerotherapist's eye' if an accident occurs while injecting under pressure. Other sclerosants used include polidocanol, popular in Germany for paravariceal injection, and absolute alcohol, while Soehandra et al (1986) have used the tissue adhesive bucrylate for large oesophageal and fundic varices.

Jensen et al (1986) compared several methods in a canine model of portal hypertension for endoscopic control of variceal bleeding, induced by puncturing a varix with a 19-gauge needle. They found sclerotherapy and the Nd:YAG laser to be most effective while the heater probe, bipolar electrocoagulation, monopolar electrocoagulation and the argon laser were relatively ineffective. They also compared sclerosing agents, and showed that 95% ethanol, 5% morrhuate, 1.5% STD and 5% ethanolamine oleate would sclerose more than 60% of veins when injected intravenously, but 95% ethanol was the most damaging with an 80% rate of severe ulceration. A combination of 1% STD, 32% ethanol and saline was effective yet with a low frequency of oesophageal damage.

Most sclerosants are detergents and animal work suggests that contact with the endothelium of the varix for only 1 second is sufficient to produce thrombosis (Dietrich and Sinapius, 1968). Transient exposure to sclerosant can therefore be effective, rendering compression devices superfluous.

There is considerable variation in the reported time interval between courses of sclerotherapy. The longer a varix remains patent and sizable, however, the more likely it is to bleed (Rose et al, 1983), so short treatment intervals are desirable. In a controlled trial of weekly versus three-weekly sclerotherapy, varices were obliterated more quickly with the shorter treatment interval with no increase in complications (Westaby et al, 1984).

Most British endoscopists try to inject the sclerosant directly into the varix, but some European workers have advocated injection into the lamina propria and submucosa alongside the varix, producing submucosal oedema which is reputed to stop bleeding and eventually to bury the varix in a protective fibrous coat (Wodak, 1960). This paravariceal technique entails multiple injections of small volumes (0.5 ml) of sclerosant alongside the varix for an approximate

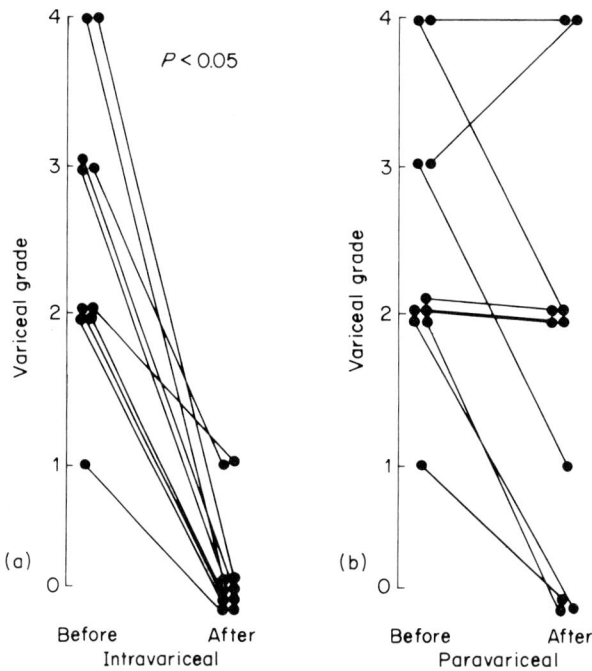

Figure 4. Results of intravariceal and paravariceal injection in two comparable groups of ten varices. Intravariceal injection was more successful at thrombosing varices ($P < 0.05$). From Rose et al (1983), *Gut* **24**, 946-9, by kind permission of the editor.

distance of 6 cm. Whatever method is used, however, most patients probably end up with a combination of intra- and paravariceal injections, particularly in the early stages when haemorrhage may obscure the varix, and later when the varix becomes small. Using a mixture of urografin and STD, 1 in 5 for large varices and 1 in 3 for small varices, intended intravariceal injections were shown radiologically to be paravariceal, although intravariceal injections were more effective at producing variceal thrombosis (Rose et al, 1983). In a similar study, 44% of attempted (Figure 4) intravariceal injections resulted in paravariceal extravasation of contrast (Grobe et al, 1984). It has also been estimated that 10–15% of paravariceal injections end up intravariceally (Conn and Grace, 1985).

Further evidence in favour of the intravascular route has come from Witzel and Wolbergs (1984), although Raschke and Paquet (1984) and The Copenhagen Esophageal Varices Sclerotherapy Project group (1984) have produced impressive results with the paravariceal route. The paravariceal technique requires a longer period of treatment and recurrent bleeding is more common before obliteration has occurred (Soehendra et al, 1983).

Complications

Bleeding is rarely precipitated by sclerotherapy, unless coughing or struggling leads to variceal laceration by the injection needle. Perforation of the oesophagus at the time of the procedure has been seen in up to 5% of injections carried out by the rigid oesophagoscope, but is rare with a fibrescope. Pulmonary aspiration of blood or other fluids in the oesophagus may complicate the procedure, although this is more common when undertaken during active variceal bleeding.

Substernal local pain is the commonest local complication and is due to tissue extravasation. It lasts for up to 48 hours, resolves quickly and responds to alkalis. Two cases of acute respiratory failure after intravariceal injection of sodium morrhuate (Monroe et al, 1983) and one of heart failure after paravariceal injection of polidocanol (Paterlini et al, 1984) have been described.

Oesophageal ulceration has been reported in 11–27% of patients (Rose and Smith, 1983). The incidence is, however, dependent upon the timing of subsequent endoscopy after sclerotherapy, as ulcers will usually heal within three weeks. In one trial in which sclerotherapy was carried out at one-week or three-week intervals, ulcers were found in 80% and 30% of cases respectively (Westaby et al, 1984). In another, Sarin et al (1986), using intravariceal absolute alcohol, found ulcers in 94% of patients at endoscopy one day later, in 69% of patients at one week and in 13% at three weeks. There was a strong correlation between the incidence of ulceration and the volume of sclerosant used, all patients who received 3 ml or more developing ulcers. The ulcers are usually painless, but may initially be associated with fever. The radiological pattern of paravariceal injections suggests that the ulcers result from sclerosant spreading along the vein sheath, ulcerating the overlying mucosa. Sometimes the ulcer may penetrate the vein wall, causing secondary haemorrhage, usually about 9–13 days after treatment. Occasionally the ulcer may penetrate the full thickness of the oesophageal wall to produce mediastinitis, fever or a pleural effusion. Perforation, oesophageal aortic fistulae and broncho-oesophageal fistulae have also been described (Carr-Locke and Sidky, 1982).

The commonest late complication of sclerotherapy is an oesophageal stricture, reported in 16–27% of patients. Whereas a single misplaced injection of sclerosant can result in oesophageal ulcer, multiple injections are required to produce sufficient fibrosis to produce a stricture. The development of a stricture fortunately coincides with the disappearance of the varices. In half of the patients, the stricture will spontaneously resolve, and in the other half it will require one or two dilatations by the Eder-Puestow technique. If no more than 2 ml of sclerosant is used for each injection, and the injections are intravariceal, strictures will rarely result.

Oesophageal studies in patients who have undergone sclerotherapy have confirmed abnormalities in oesophageal motility with a reduced percentage of peristaltic contractions. Acid reflux (Reilly et al, 1984) and reduction in lower oesophageal sphincter pressure (Ogle et al, 1978) have been found in single studies but have not been confirmed in others (Soderlund and Thor, 1985). Symptomatic disturbances in oesophageal motor function after sclerotherapy are rarely met with.

The mortality of sclerotherapy is very low (about 1%), often following mediastinitis or perforation, but the long-term outlook depends on hepatic function, which is usually poor in cirrhotics.

Bacteraemia has been looked for during sclerotherapy. It is transient, does not lead to sepsis (Sauerbruch et al, 1985), and was found to be due to contamination of the endoscopic water bottle in one centre (Brayko et al, 1985), from where it was easily eliminated.

One interesting long-term effect of sclerotherapy is on the radiological appearance of the oesophagus. Fifteen patients, whose oesophageal varices had been obliterated, were examined by double contrast barium swallow. In nine (60%) the oesophagus was abnormal, demonstrating sharp-edged longitudinal tramline filling defects and an irregular, patchy nodularity with loss of the normal longitudinal folds. These appearances represented redundant epithelial folds, epithelial tags and healed ulcers (Rose et al, 1985).

Randomised trials of sclerotherapy

The first reported controlled trial of sclerotherapy came from Cape Town (Terblanche et al, 1979). Survival and the recurrence rates of variceal haemorrhage were compared in a group treated by intravariceal endoscopic sclerotherapy using a rigid endoscope under general anaesthesia with another group treated by orthodox medical therapy, but also, for ethical reasons, with acute sclerotherapy if active variceal bleeding was diagnosed. The treatment group had fewer bleeds than the control group, although a follow-up publication in 1983 (Terblanche et al, 1983) found that mortality was the same in the two groups despite the reduced incidence of bleeding in the treated patients. However, 37% of the control group had partial or complete obliteration of their varices—an obvious distorting factor.

The King's College Hospital trial (Westaby et al, 1985b) was the first to show a reduction in mortality with sclerotherapy. Only five patients out of 56 died from bleeding after intravenous sclerotherapy during a mean follow-up period of 37 months, whereas 25 out of 60 patients in the control group died of variceal haemorrhage, a highly significant difference ($P < 0.001$). Sclerotherapy reduced the overall bleeding rate per patient-month threefold, and the great majority of haemorrhages occurred before the varices had been obliterated. Over four years, survival was significantly greater in the sclerotherapy group (60%) than in the control group (31%; $P < 0.001$). Ten treated patients died from liver failure and one from a hepatoma, however, as the underlying cirrhosis remained a problem.

The Copenhagen Esophageal Varices Sclerotherapy Project published its findings in 1984; 187 unselected patients with cirrhosis were randomly assigned to medical treatment or to paravariceal sclerotherapy and were followed for up to 52 months. During this time, 65% of the sclerotherapy group and 78% of the control group died. Most of the deaths occurred in the first two months while the varices were still present; thereafter, the mortality declined to only 43% of the untreated group.

The Los Angeles sclerotherapy trial (Korula et al, 1985) failed to show an improvement in the survival of the treated group, but 21% of patients were lost to follow-up, and in only 28 of the original treatment group of 63 was variceal obliteration achieved. The trial did confirm a reduction in rebleeding in the sclerotherapy group, however, and if the patients undergoing shunt surgery were withdrawn from analysis, there was a significant difference in survival in favour of the treated group.

All four trials thus show a significant reduction in the total number of bleeding episodes with sclerotherapy. They also demonstrate the frequency of further haemorrhage within the first two or three months of treatment, prior to variceal obliteration. Such episodes were seldom life threatening, but the addition of propranolol to the treatment regimen prior to the disappearance of the varices had no effect on the frequency of recurrent variceal bleeding (Westaby et al, 1986).

There have been two trials to compare sclerotherapy with Sengstaken-Blakemore tube tamponade in controlling acute variceal haemorrhage. Barsoum et al (1982) were able to control the acute bleeding episode in 74% by sclerotherapy and in 42% by balloon tamponade, a significant difference. A similar study from Germany (Paquet and Feussner, 1985) achieved control of active bleeding in 19 out of 21 patients (91%) managed by sclerotherapy. In comparison, balloon tamponade controlled bleeding in significantly fewer patients—12 (55%) of 22 patients. The mortality was improved in Paquet's but not in the Egyptian study.

There have been a number of other small published trials of sclerotherapy, and almost all have confirmed that it is more effective than medical treatment alone, whether the injections are intravariceal or paravariceal. Sclerotherapy has become the treatment of choice, but for the actively bleeding patient who is not controlled by a Sengstaken tube, it often proves impracticable, and anastomotic gun transection of the oesophagus may be life saving (Johnston, 1982). In a comparison of transection with sclerotherapy, similar death rates were found (16/39 vs 15/37). There were 11 deaths from rebleeding and three from liver failure in the sclerotherapy group, however, and whereas no deaths from rebleeding occurred in the transection group, nine patients died of liver failure (Huinzinga et al, 1985).

Prophylactic sclerotherapy

Injection sclerotherapy for patients with large varices who have not previously bled is controversial. Paquet (1982) performed a controlled trial and found that during three years of follow-up 29 (87%) of the control patients had a variceal bleed and 21 (64%) died. After sclerotherapy only three (9%) patients bled and only six (19%) died. Another German trial (Witzel and Wolbergs, 1985) has also confirmed the place of prophylactic sclerotherapy, but both these trials are characterised by a much higher rate of variceal bleeding in the control group than would be expected in Britain for alcoholic cirrhosis, which may give bias to the results. A third, more recent German study (Koch et al, 1986) has failed to show a decline in mortality with prophylactic sclerotherapy, 33% of the control group and 37% of the treated group dying over a mean follow-up period of 36 months. The most frequent cause of death was variceal bleeding in the control group and liver failure in the treated group. Three patients developed a mucosal ulcer after sclerotherapy that led to haemorrhage requiring transfusion, three had an oesophageal stricture and one each developed an empyema and a pleural effusion.

At present, prophylactic for large varices is justified only in controlled clinical trials (Terblanche, 1986). For small varices the risk of bleeding is slight, the chance of extravasation of sclerosant is increased and complications are common. They should therefore be left alone.

Follow-up

162 patients whose varices had been obliterated by sclerotherapy were followed up for periods of up to six years. New varices developed in 99 and were a cause of bleeding in 28, of whom 3 died. Almost all recurrences took place within the first year of follow-up (Westaby and Williams, 1984). Similar results were obtained in Cardiff, where 50 patients were followed up for two years after eradication of oesophageal varices (Rose and Smith, 1984). Varices recurred in 20, 17 of which were diagnosed within the first year of follow-up. Only three patients bled from these varices, however. As sclerotherapy does not affect the underlying live disease, it was not surprising that 13 (26%) died during follow-up, seven of hepatic failure, three from infection, two from non-variceal bleeding and one from a hepatoma.

Based on these results, it is important to follow patients after variceal obliteration, at three-monthly intervals for the first year, six-monthly intervals for the second year and, if no recurrence has occurred, annually therafter.

Summary

Injection sclerotherapy is the best available treatment for bleeding varices. Unlike the portacaval shunt, it does not produce encephalopathy and does not require general anaesthesia. Controlled trials have shown the technique to significantly reduce the risk of variceal bleeding, and in two of them to reduce the mortality. In the first few weeks, however, when the varices are still large, the rebleeding risk remains high. Once the varices have been obliterated, death from variceal haemorrhage is most unlikely although the underlying cause of the liver disease will also require treatment, and death from liver failure and hepatomas will continue to occur.

Injection sclerotherapy is not the only treatment for oesophageal varices. Balloon tamponade and vasoconstrictor drugs are very useful in the management of the acute bleeder, and oesophageal transection with the anastomotic gun may be life saving in the early stages before sclerotherapy becomes effective. Varices recur after transection, however, and long-term endoscopic follow-up will be required.

The place of long-term propranolol to lessen the risk of variceal bleeding remains controversial, and until further controlled trials are completed, propranolol cannot be recommended.

References

Barsoum MS, Boulas FI, El-Rooby AA, Rizk-Allah MA and Ibrahim AS (1982) Tamponade and injection sclerotherapy in the management of bleeding oesophageal varices. *Br. J. Surg.* **69**, 76–8.

Blenkinsopp WK (1968) Comparison of tetradecylsulphate of sodium with other sclerosants in rats. *Br. J. Exp. Pathol.* **49**, 197–201.

Brayko CM, Kozarek RA, Sanowski RA and Testa AW (1985) Bacteraemia during oesophageal variceal sclerotherapy: its cause and prevention. *Gastrointest. Endosc.* **31**, 10–12.

Burroughs AK, Jenkins WJ, Sherlock S et al (1983) Controlled trial of propranolol for the prevention of recurrent variceal hemorrhage in patients with cirrhosis. *N. Engl. J. Med.* **309**, 1539–42.

Carr-Locke DL and Sidky K (1982) Broncho-oesophageal fistula: a late complication of endoscopic variceal sclerotherapy. *Gut* **23**, 1005–07.

Clanet J, Tournut R, Fourtanier G, Joncquiert F and Pascal JP (1978) Traitement por la pitressine des hémorragies par rupture de varices oesophagiennes chez le cirrhotique. Étude controlée. *Acta Gastroenterol. Belg.* **41**, 539–43.

Conn HO (1984) Propranolol in portal hypertension—problems in paradise? *Hepatology* **4**, 560–4.

Conn HO and Grace ND (1985) Portal hypertension and sclerotherapy of oesophageal varices. A point of view. *Endosc. Rev.* **2**, 39–53.

Conn HO and Lindenmuth WW (1968) Prophylactic portacaval anastomosis in cirrhotic patients with oesophageal varices. *N. Engl. J. Med.* **279**, 725–32.

Crafoord C and Frenckner P (1939) New surgical treatment of varicose veins of the oesophagus. *Acta Otolaryngol. (Stockholm)* **27**, 422–9.

De Carvalho AF (1966) Sur l'angio-architecture veinuse de la zone de transition oesophago-gastrique et son interprétation fonctionelle. *Acta Anat.* **64**, 125–62.

Dick R (1981) Transhepatic injection of varices. *Brit. J. Hosp. Med.* **26**, 340–47.

Dietrich HP and Sinapius D (1968) Esperimentelle Endothelschadingung durch Varizenverodungsmittel. *Arzneimittelforsch* **18**, 116–20.

Fleischer D (1985) Endoscopic ND: YAG laser therapy for active oesophageal variceal bleeding. *Gastrointest. Endosc.* **31**, 4–9.

Freeman JG, Cobden I, Lishman AH and Record CO (1982) Controlled trial of terlipressin (glypressin) versus vasopressin in the early treatment of oesophageal varices. *Lancet* **ii**, 66–8.

Gimson AES, Westaby D, Hegarty J, Watson A and Williams R (1986) A randomised trial of vasopressin and vasopressin plus Nitroglycerin in the control of acute variceal haemorrhage. *Hepatology* **6**, 410–13.

Grobe JL, Kozarek RA, Sanowski RA, Legrand J and Kovac A (1984) Venography during endoscopic injection sclerotherapy of esophageal varices. *Gastrointest. Endosc.* **30**, 6–8.

Hamilton G, Jenkins WM, Burroughs A, McIntyre N and Hobbs KEF (1984) Oesophageal transaction for variceal bleeding. *Lancet* **i**, 219–20.

Harley HAJ, Morgan T, Redeker AG et al (1986) Results of a randomised trial of end-to-side portacaval shunt and distal splenoranal shunt in alcoholic liver disease and variceal bleeding. *Gastroenterology* **91**, 802–9.

Huizinga WKJ, Angorn IB and Baker LW (1985) Esophageal transection versus injection sclerotherapy in the management of bleeding esophageal varices in patients at high risk. *Surg. Gynecol. Obstet.* **160**, 539–46.

Hussey KP (1985) Vasopressin therapy for upper gastrointestinal tract hemorrhage. Has its efficacy been proven? *Arch. Intern. Med.* **145**, 1263–67.

Jenkins SA, Baxter JN, Corbett W et al (1985) A prospective randomised controlled clinical trial comparing somatostatin and vasopressin in controlling acute variceal haemorrhage. *Br. Med. J.* **290**, 275–7.

Jensen DM, Machicado GA and Silpa M (1986) Esophageal varix hemorrhage and sclerotherapy-animal studies. *Endoscopy* **18** (Suppl. 2): 18–22.

Johnston GW (1982) Six years' experience of oesophageal transection for oesophageal varices using a circular stapling gun. *Gut* **23**, 770–73.

Kiefhaber P, Kiefhaber K, Huber F and Nash G (1983) Usefulness of Nd:YAG laser applications in acute gastrointestinal haemorrhage. *Laser Surg. Med.* **3**, 111–13.

Kitano S, Terblanche J, Kahn D and Bornman PC (1986) Venous anatomy of the lower oesophagus in portal hypertension: practical implications. *Br. J. Surg.* **73**, 525–31.

Koch H, Henning H, Grimm H and Soehendra H (1986) Prophylactic sclerosing of esophageal varices—results of a prospective controlled study. *Endoscopy* **18**, 40–3.

Korula J, Balart LA, Radvan G et al (1985) A prospective randomized controlled trial of chronic esophageal variceal sclerotherapy. *Hepatology* **5**, 584–89.

Lebrec D, De Fleury P, Rueff B, Nahum H and Benhamou JP (1980a). Portal hypertension, size of esophageal varices and risk of gastrointestinal bleeding in alcoholic cirrhosis. *Gastroenterology* **179**, 1139–44.

Lebrec D, Nouel O, Corbic M and Benhamou JP (1980b) Propranolol—a medical treatment for portal hypertension. *Lancet* **ii**, 180–2.

Lebrec D, Poynard T, Bernuau J et al (1984) A randomised controlled study of propranolol for prevention of recurrent gastrointestinal bleeding in patients with cirrhosis: a final report. *Hepatology* **4**, 355–8.

Lunderquist A and Vang J (1974) Transhepatic catheterization and obliteration of the coronary vein in patients with portal hypertension and esophageal varices. *N. Engl. J. Med.* **291**, 646–9.

Macbeth R (1955) Treatment of oesophageal varices in portal hypertension by means of sclerosing injections. *Br. Med. J.* **2**, 877–80.

McCormack TT, Rose JD, Smith PM and Johnson AG (1983) Perforating veins and blood flow in oesophageal varices. *Lancet* **ii**, 1442–4.

Maillard JN, Rueff B, Prandic D, Sicot C (1974) Hepatic arterialization and portacaval shunt in hepatic cirrhosis. An assessment. *Arch. Surg.* **108**, 315–20.

Merigan TC Jr, Plotkim GR and Davidson CS (1962) The effect of intravenous pituitrin on haemorrhage from bleeding esophageal varices. A controlled evaluation. *N. Engl. J. Med.* **266**, 134–7.

Monroe P, Morrow CF Jr, Millen JE, Fairman RP and Glauser FL (1983) Acute respiratory failure after sodium morrhuate and esophageal sclerotherapy. *Gastroenterology* **85**, 693–9.

Noda T (1984) Angioarchitectural study of esophageal varices. *Virchows Arch. (Pathol. Anat.)* **404**, 381–92.

Ogle SJ, Kirk CJC, Bailey RJ et al (1978) Esophageal function in cirrhotic patients undergoing injection sclerotherapy for oesophageal varices. *Digestion* **18**, 178–85.

Osborne DR and Hobbs KEF (1981) The acute treatment of haemorrhage from oesophageal varices: a comparison of oesophageal transection and staple gun anastomosis with portacaval shunt. *Br. J. Surg.* **68**, 734–7.

Paquet KJ (1982) Prophylactic endoscopic treatment of the oesophageal wall in varices—a prospective controlled randomised trial. *Endoscopy* **14**, 4–5.

Paquet KH and Feussner H (1985) Endoscopic sclerosis and esophageal tamponade in acute haemorrhage from esophagogastric varices. A prospective controlled randomized trial. *Hepatology* **5**, 580–3.

Paterlini A, Salmi A, Buffoli F and Lombardi C (1984) Heart failure and endoscopic sclerotherapy of variceal bleeding. *Lancet* i, 1241.

Pinto Correia P, Alves MM, Alexandrino P, Silveira J (1984) Controlled trial of vasopressin and balloon tamponade in bleeding esophageal varices. *Hepatology* **4**, 885–8.

Price JB Jr, Voorhees AB Jr and Britton RC (1967) Operative hemodynamics in portal hypertension. *Arch. Surg.* **95**, 843–9.

Raptis S and Zoupas C (1979) Somatostatin not helpful in bleeding esophageal varices. *N. Engl. J. Med.* **300**, 739.

Raschke E and Paquet KT (1984) Management of haemorrhage from esophageal varices using the esophagoscopic sclerosing method. *Ann. Surg.* **177**, 99–102.

Reilly JJ, Schade RR and Van Thiel DS (1984) Esophageal function after injection sclerotherapy. Pathogenesis of esophageal stricture. *Am. J. Surg.* **147**, 85–8.

Resnick RH, Iber FL, Ishihara AM, Chalmers TC, Zimmerman H (1974) A controlled study of the therapeutic portacaval shunt. *Gastroenterology* **67**, 843–57.

Rose JDR and Smith PM (1983) Natural history of endoscopic oesophageal sclerotherapy complications. *Gut* **24**, A1003.

Rose JDR and Smith PM (1984) Factors affecting variceal recurrence after endoscopic sclerotherapy. *Gut* **25**, A577.

Rose JDR, Crane MD and Smith PM (1983) Factors affecting successful endoscopic sclerotherapy for oesophageal varices. *Gut* **24**, 946–9.

Rose JDR, Roberts GM and Smith PM (1985) The radiological appearances of the oesophagus after sclerotherapy for varices. *Clin. Radiol.* **36**, 355–8.

Rueff B, Prandi B, Degos F et al (1976) A controlled study of therapeutic portacaval shunt in alcoholic cirrhosis. *Lancet* i, 655–9.

Sarin SK and Nundy S (1984) Balloon tamponade in the management of bleeding oesophageal varices. *Ann. Roy. Coll. Surg.* **66**, 30–2.

Sarin SK, Nanda R, Vij JC and Anand BS (1986) Oseophageal ulceration after sclerotherapy—a complication or an accompaniment? *Endoscopy* **18**, 44–5.

Sauerbruch T, Holl J, Ruckdeschel G, Forsti J and Weinzerl M (1985) Bacteraemia associated with endoscopic sclerotherapy of oesophageal varices. *Endoscopy* **17**, 170–2.

Silk DBA et al (1979) In Williams R and Cantani I (eds) *Recenti Progressi in Epatologi*, pp 5–12. Milan: Ambrosiano.

Soderlund C and Thor K (1985) Esophageal function after sclerotherapy for bleeding varices. *Acta Chir. Scand. Suppl.* **524**, 63–1.

Soehendra N, de Heer K, Kempeneers I and Frommelt L (1983) Morphological alterations of the esophagus after endoscopic sclerotherapy of varices. *Endoscopy* **15**, 291–6.

Soehendra N, Nam VCh, Grimm H and Kempeneers I (1986) Endoscopic obliteration of large oesophagogastric varices with bucrylate. *Endoscopy* **18**, 25–26.

Sonnenberg GE, Keller V, Perruchoud A, Burckhardt D and Gyr K (1981) Effect of somatostatin on splanchnic hemodynamics in patients with cirrhosis of the liver and in normal subjects. *Gastroenterology* **80**, 526–30.

Spence RAJ, Anderson JR and Johnston GW (1985) Twenty five years of injection sclerotherapy for bleeding varices. *Br. J. Surg.* **72**, 195–8.

Sugiura M and Futagawa S (1984) Esophageal transection with paraesophagogastric devascularizations (the Sugiura procedure) in the treatment of esophageal varices. *World J. Surg.* **8**, 673–82.

Terblanche J (1986) Sclerotherapy for prophylaxis of variceal bleeding. *Lancet* i, 961–3.

Terblanche J, Northover JMA, Bornman P et al (1979) A prospective controlled trial of sclerotherapy in the long term management of patients after esophageal variceal bleeding. *Surg. Gynecol. Obstet.* **148**, 323–3.

Terblanche J, Bornman PC, Kahn D et al (1983) Failure of repeated injection sclerotherapy to improve long term survival after oesophageal variceal bleeding. A five year prospective controlled trial. *Lancet* **2**, 1328–32.

Teres J, Anastasio C, Bordas JM et al (1978) Esophageal tamponade for bleeding varices. Controlled trial between the Sengstaken-Blakemore tube and the Linton-Nicholas tube. *Gastroenterology* **75**, 566–9.

Teres J, Bordas JM, Bravo MD, Visa J, Pera C and Rhodes J (1986) Endoscopic sclerotherapy vs distal splenorenal shunt in the elective treatment of variceal haemorrhage. A randomized controlled trial. *J. Hepatol. Suppl. I* 3, 525.

The Copenhagen Esophageal Varices Sclerotherapy Project (1984) Sclerotherapy after first variceal haemorrhage in cirrhosis. A randomised multicenter trial. *N. Engl. J. Med.* **311**, 1594–1600.

Thulin L, Tyden G, Samnegard H, Muhrbeck O and Efendie S (1979) Treatment of bleeding oesophageal varices with somatostatin. *Acta Chir. Scand.* **145**, 395–9.

Trudeau W and Prindiville T (1986) Endoscopic injection sclerosis in bleeding gastric varices. *Gastrointest. Endosc.* **32**, 264–8.

Tyden G, Samnegard H, Thulin L, Friman L and Efendie S (1978) Treatment of bleeding esophageal varices with somatostatin. *N. Engl. J. Med.* **299**, 1466–8.

Walker RM (1964) Oesophageal transection for bleeding varices. *Surg. Gynec. Obstet.* **118**, 323–9.

Warren WD, Zeppa R and Fomon JJ (1967) Selective transplenic decompression of gastroesophageal varices by distal splenorenal shunt. *Ann. Surg.* **166**, 437–55.

Warren WD, Salam AA, Hutson D and Zeppa R (1974) Selective distal splenorenal shunt: technique and results of operation. *Arch. Surg.* **108**, 306–14.

Warren WD, Galambos JT, Riepe SP et al (1986) Distal splenorenal shunt versus endoscopic sclerotherapy for long term management of variceal bleeding. Preliminary report of a prospective randomized trial. *Ann. Surg.* **203**, 454–63.

Westaby D and Williams R (1984) Follow up study after sclerotherapy. *Scand. J. Gastroenterol.* **19** (Suppl. 102), 71–5.

Westaby D, Melia WM, Macdougall BRD, Hegarty JE and Williams R (1984) Injection sclerotherapy for oesophageal varices: a prospective randomized trial of different treatment schedules. *Gut* **25**, 129–32.

Westaby D, Melia WM, Macdougall BRD et al (1985a) B$_1$ selective adrenoreceptor blockade for the long term management of variceal bleeding. A prospective randomized trial to compare oral metoprolol with injection sclerotherapy in cirrhosis. *Gut* **26**, 421–5.

Westaby D, Macdougall BRD and Williams R (1985b) Improved survival following injection sclerotherapy for esophageal varices: final analysis of a controlled trial. *Hepatology* **5**, 827–30.

Westaby D, Melia W, Hegarty JE et al (1986) Use of propranolol to reduce the rebleeding rate during injection sclerotherapy prior to variceal obliteration. *Hepatology* **6**, 673–5.

Witzel L and Wolbergs E (1985) Prospektive Kontrollierte Studie einer para- und intravarikösen Verödungs—therapie bein Ösophagusvarizen. *Schweiz. Med. Wochenschr.* **114**, 599–601.

Wodak E (1960) Ösophagusvarizen blunting bei portaler Hypertension: Ihr Therapie und Prophylaxe. *Wien Med. Wochenschr.* **110**, 581–3.

Key Developments in Gastroenterology
Edited by P. R. Salmon
© 1988 John Wiley & Sons Ltd

3

Liver Transplantation

Roger Williams
Rex J. Polson
King's College Hospital and School of Medicine and Dentistry, Denmark Hill, London

Introduction

The first human liver transplant was carried out by Starzl in 1963, and the first liver graft of the Cambridge/King's College Hospital series was performed by Calne in 1968. Two other groups with considerable early experience in this field were Krom in Groningen and Pichlmayr in Hannover. The data given by these groups, and by the other participants in the National Institutes of Health Consensus Development Conference (NIHCDC) in 1983, led to the following conclusion: 'Liver transplantation is a therapeutic modality for end-stage liver disease that deserves broader application' (NIHCDC Statement, 1984). This has been followed by a very rapid increase in the number of centres in America and Europe which have either initiated or are planning programmes as well as marked expansion in the already established transplant programmes. Consequently there has been an exponential increase in the number of patients receiving orthotopic liver transplants in Europe and the USA as well as in Great Britain (Figure 1).

This increase in the number of patients transplanted in our programme has been dependent on an equally rapid rise in the number of donor organs offered to our liver transplant co-ordinator between 1982 and 1986 (Table 1). Since 1984 there has also been a considerable increase in the number of organs offered in the paediatric age group. This is in part explained by a popular television programme which became involved in the plight of one of our young children with biliary atresia and the need for transplant facilities for infants and children in the UK. This led to an enormous increase in the general public's awareness of liver transplantation and in many instances since then, the request for organs to be used for liver grafting has come from the families of those dying. At the same time, doctors in general have been urged to take a more positive attitude to the potential use of organs from patients dying from accidents or other causes.

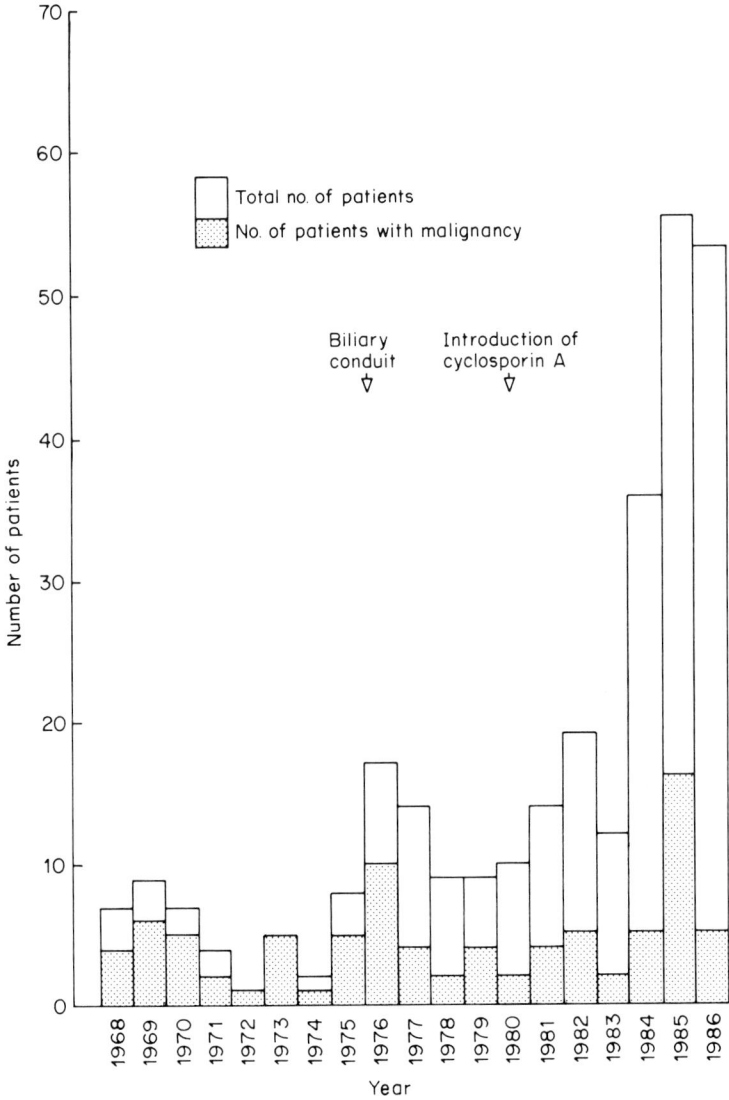

Figure 1. Increase in the number of patients in the UK undergoing orthotopic liver transplantation and the proportion each year with hepatic malignancy.

Patient Selection and Pretransplant Assessment

Liver grafting should be considered for any patient with a progressive or otherwise fatal liver disorder who is no longer able to live a reasonable existence but is still well enough to withstand the major surgery involved. The

Table 1. Increase in the number of donor organs offered to the Cambridge/King's College Hospital transplant programme following media publicity in January 1984.

Year	Total	Within UK	Abroad
1982	45	33	12
1983	96	52	44
1984	225	187	38
1985	267	241	26
1 Dec. 1986	384	–	–

Cambridge/King's College Hospital series, like most other transplant programmes, includes almost every type of end-stage liver disease (Table 2). In practice, the decisions as to which patients should be treated and when can be very difficult.

In children, particularly those aged two years or less, liver transplantation is accompanied by a greater number of technical difficulties often related to congenital anomalies. In addition it is essential that the size of the donor organ be matched carefully to the size of the donor, so that vascular insufficiency and hepatic infarction are avoided. Although Starzl's results have always been better in children than in adults, until recently we had performed few liver transplants in children because, until the advent of cyclosporin A, we were concerned about the long-term effects of corticosteroids, particularly retardation of growth and osteoporosis. Older age is, however, less of a bar than previously, and although cardiorespiratory complications become increasingly common over the age of 40 years, most transplant series, as in ours, include occasional patients in their 60s.

Table 2. Indications for liver transplantation in the Cambridge/King's College Hospital series (May 1968–26 November 1986).

Primary liver tumour		68	Cirrhosis		156
Hepatocellular carcinoma	51		Primary biliary	58	
Intrahepatic cholangiocarcinoma	13		CAH/Cirrhosis	54	
Sarcoma	4		Alcoholic	7	
			Sclerosing cholangitis/		
			secondary biliary	19	
Carcinoma of hepatic ducts		10	α_1-Antitrypsin deficiency	7	
			Wilson's disease	4	
Hepatic metastases		6			
			Other metabolic	7	
Apudoma/carcinoid		3			
			Budd-Chiari syndrome		17
			Acute/subacute liver failure		16
			Biliary atresia/neonatal hepatitis		22
			Polycystic liver		2

Total = 300

Indeed Starzl has recently carried out a liver transplant in a 76-year-old-woman with primary biliary cirrhosis and she left hospital well three weeks later. In spite of this, those patients with major limitations of cardiac or respiratory function will need excluding.

The risks of liver grafting are considerably greater in patients with portal hypertension if they have had previous upper abdominal surgery, as this greatly increases the hazards of dissection and the likely blood loss.

Intraoperative blood usage is also closely correlated to the severity of the pre-operative coagulation abnormality (Bontempo et al, 1985) and, not surprisingly, blood usage and survival are inversely related. Indeed in a recent report, the survival rate for adult patients receiving up to 30 units of blood was 70%, while for patients who required more than 30 units survival was only 14% (Van Thiel et al, 1986). Starzl's group have found that the small shrunken liver, which is commonly present in long-standing cirrhosis, is often technically difficult to replace and is associated with a poor prognosis; our own experience would support this. Poor nutrition and muscle wasting in patients with chronic parenchymatous liver disease are further adverse factors which often result in reduced resistance to infection postoperatively. Stringent efforts must therefore be made to eradicate any preoperative infection in these patients, before exposure to the added risks of immunosuppression.

In a recent study the preoperative serum creatinine level has been shown to be the best indicator of short-term prognosis after liver transplantation, with levels either less than or greater than $147.4\,\mu$mol/l (1.72 mg/dl) accurately predicting survival or death, respectively, in 79% of cases (Cuervas-Mons et al, 1986). Other variables that were associated with a significant risk of death were ascites, hepatic encephalopathy, elevated white blood and polymorphonuclear cell count, decreased helper to suppressor T-cell ratio and elevated bilirubin levels. It has also been suggested that thyroid hormone levels, particularly rT_3 levels, might be helpful in predicting the likely prognosis in patients awaiting liver grafting (Van Thiel et al, 1985). Those with higher levels of rT_3 had a very poor prognosis while those with high T_4 and low T_3 levels appeared to have a better chance of survival both up to and after liver transplantation.

Malignant liver disease

All published experience points to a significant risk of tumour recurrence and indeed in our programme between 45 and 100% of patients who survive more than three months after transplantation have evidence of recurrence depending on the tumour type (Table 3). In spite of the many methods now available for detection of extrahepatic spread prior to transplantation, including thoracic and abdominal CT scans, lymphangiography and radioisotope bone scan, small tumour deposits may still be missed. When Mittal and colleagues (1984) compared the accuracy of preoperative CT scan with gross pathological

Table 3. Tumour recurrence in patients with hepatic malignancy treated by liver transplantation (May 1968–26 November 1986).

	Hepatoma	Cholangiocarcinoma	Sarcoma/metastases
Patients treated	51	23	10
Alive at 3 months	34	10	3
Recurrence in patients living > 3 months	45%	67%	100%

examination of the resected specimen, they found that between 20 and 47% of the various patient groups had tumour nodules evident macroscopically within the liver that were not apparent on the scan.

Nevertheless, some patients with tumours are suitable for treatment by liver transplantation which may even be curative. Our longest survivor remains well almost 11 years after his transplant which followed detection of an asymptomatic hepatocellur carcinoma in a mildly fibrotic liver as a result of familial HBsAg infection. Patients with long-standing cirrhosis in whom hepatoma development is detected at a presymptomatic stage by ultrasound or α -fetoprotein screening are a group worth considering, as are the younger patients with primary hepatocellular carcinoma in a non-cirrhotic liver, whose general condition is good and who have a relatively slow growing lesion of the fibrolamellar type, which tends to metastasise late.

Chronic end-stage liver disease

Most patients within this category have end-stage cirrhosis from chronic active hepatitis, cirrhosis of the cryptogenic variety or biliary cirrhosis (Table 2). In the latter patients the relief of pruritus, deep jaundice and pigmentation following transplantation is remarkable. Patients with chronic encephalopathy in association with a large spontaneous or surgically induced (shunt) collateral circulation and inactive liver disease, who are poorly controlled by dietary restriction and lactulose therapy, represent a small group of patients who can also show a dramatic response to successful transplantation. For the cirrhotic patient with recurrent variceal haemorrhage in whom all other measures have been tried, liver grafting may also be a life-saving procedure.

Bypass procedures, which decompress the inferior vena cava and portal vein and so reduce the accumulation of potassium and acid waste products while also helping to maintain blood pressure and tissue perfusion, have been used to differing degrees in these patients with cirrhosis. Thus, venovenous bypass (Shaw et al, 1984) is used in nearly all adult patients by Starzl and colleagues, while in the Cambridge/King's College Hospital series bypass is used in only 10% of cases and venoarterial bypass is the method employed (Calne et al, 1984).

The decision as to when liver grafting should be performed in patients with cirrhosis will be dependent on both clinical and biochemical criteria. For patients with primary biliary cirrhosis (PBC) it has been shown that once the serum bilirubin has exceeded 100 μmol/l the prognosis is usually less than two years and a prognostic index based on six independent variables has recently been developed (Neuberger et al, 1986).

In several of these conditions there have been reports of recurrence of the disorder in the grafted liver some time after successful transplantation. Thus, mild recurrence of the PBC has been reported in several patients who have survived for three or more years (Neuberger et al, 1982) and although Fennel et al (1983) have suggested that such changes in liver histology are the consequence of continuing rejection, in our experience they are quite distinct. In autoimmune chronic active hepatitis where, as in PBC, immune mechanisms play a major role in pathogenesis, recurrence of the disease might also be anticipated and we have recently reported this in a 21-year-old-woman who had a liver transplant in 1980 (Neuberger et al, 1984).

Patients who are HBsAg- and HBeAg-positive in whom active viral replication is continuing, should not be transplanted owing to the risk of infection of the donor liver by hepatitis B virus. Four patients treated early in our series were given high titre immunoglobulin at the time of surgery and this appeared to be effective in clearing the circulation of HBsAg, although subsequent testing of stored sera from these patients revealed that all were HBeAb-positive. From recent reports of the use of liver transplantation in patients with presumed non-A, non-B virus, it appears that this too may infect the donor liver in the early postoperative period and result in a severe hepatitis which can be fatal (Wall et al, 1985).

In the severe cases of Budd–Chiari syndrome, liver transplantation probably carries less risk overall than a side-to-side shunt whilst also offering the chance of a complete cure. As these patients may well have a primary coagulation abnormality, there is a significant risk of recurrent thrombosis after liver grafting. Thus of the 17 patients with Budd–Chiari syndrome treated in the Cambridge/King's College Hospital series, seven have developed vascular

Table 4. Inborn errors of metabolism that have been treated by liver transplantation.

Liver severely damaged and other organs affected	Other organs primarily affected
α_1-Antitrypsin deficiency	Primary hyperoxaluria
Wilson's disease	Crigler-Najjar syndrome
Protoporphyria	Primary hypercholesterolaemia
Tyrosinosis	Neimann-Pick disease
Galactosaemia	Sea blue histocyte syndrome
Glycogen storage disease	
Bylers disease	

thromboses after transplantation, and in six this occurred in spite of treatment with anticoagulants. However, it is now nine years since our longest survivor was transplanted for this condition and the actual one-year survival for the whole group is 77%.

The number of patients with alcoholic cirrhosis who will prove suitable candidates for transplantation is likely to be small. Not only is the heavy use of alcohol associated with cardiac and cerebral impairment which, in addition to malnutrition, will add to the hazards of the operation, but also there is always the risk of a return to previous drinking habits, and possible non-compliance with drug treatment postoperatively.

Inborn errors of metabolism

Many of these disorders, which would otherwise have proved fatal, have now been successfully treated by liver transplantation. In some, the liver is not only the site of the metabolic defect but is also one of the major organs damaged, whilst in other conditions extrahepatic organs are primarily affected (Table 4). In patients with α_1-antitrypsin deficiency following liver transplantation the α_1-antitrypsin phenotype becomes that of the donor and enzyme levels are returned to normal (Table 5), whilst in patients with Wilson's disease not only are the parameters of copper metabolism restored to normal (Figure 2) but also severe neurological impairment and hepatic failure, when present, can be reversed. A 13-year-old boy with erythropoietic protoporphyria, who developed rapidly progressive cholastic jaundice earlier this year, was treated by liver transplantation and subsequently his photosensitive skin rash has resolved with a return towards normal of his porphyrin metabolism (Figure 3). In conditions affecting organs other than the liver, combined organ transplants may be required. These include combined liver and kidney transplants, which we have

Table 5. Effects of liver transplantation on patients with α_1-antitrypsin deficiency.

OL	Age/	Sex	Preoperative		Postoperative	
			Phenotype	α_1-antitrypsin level (g/l)	Phenotype	α_1-antitrypsin level (g/l)
70	16	M	PiZZ	NOT DETECTED	–	–
146	57	M	–	0.15	–	–
160	14	F	PiZZ	< 0.40	PiMS	2.7
178	5	M	PiZZ	< 0.40	–	–
181	4	F	PiZZ	0.40	PiMM	2.8
202	3	F	PiZZ/ZO	< 0.40	PiMM	Awaited
				(N.R. 1.8–3.0)		

(1 Sept. 1985)

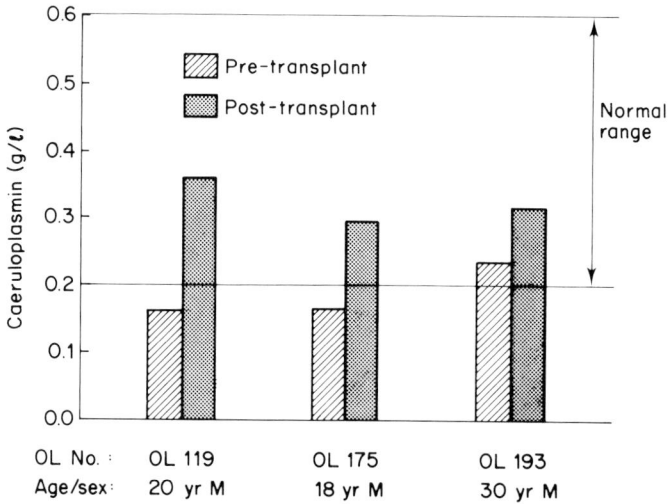

Figure 2. Effect of liver transplantation on caeruloplasmin concentration in three patients with Wilson's disease.

carried out in three patients with renal failure due to primary hyperoxaluria and which resulted in correction of the abnormal oxalate metabolic pool (Watts et al, 1985); and a combined heart and liver transplant for a young patient with

Table 6. Results of liver transplantation and fulminant hepatic failure in Cambridge/King's College Hospital series.

	Number	Survival
Fulminant hepatic failure		
3 NANB hepatitis		
1 hepatitis A		
1 drug reaction	7	42.9%
1 Wilson's disease		
1 Budd–Chiari syndrome		
Late onset hepatic failure		
4 NANB hepatitis	6	66.7%
2 drug reaction		
* *Severe acute hepatitis*		
2 NANB hepatitis	2	100.0%

* Long history
+ Coagulopathy but no encephalopathy

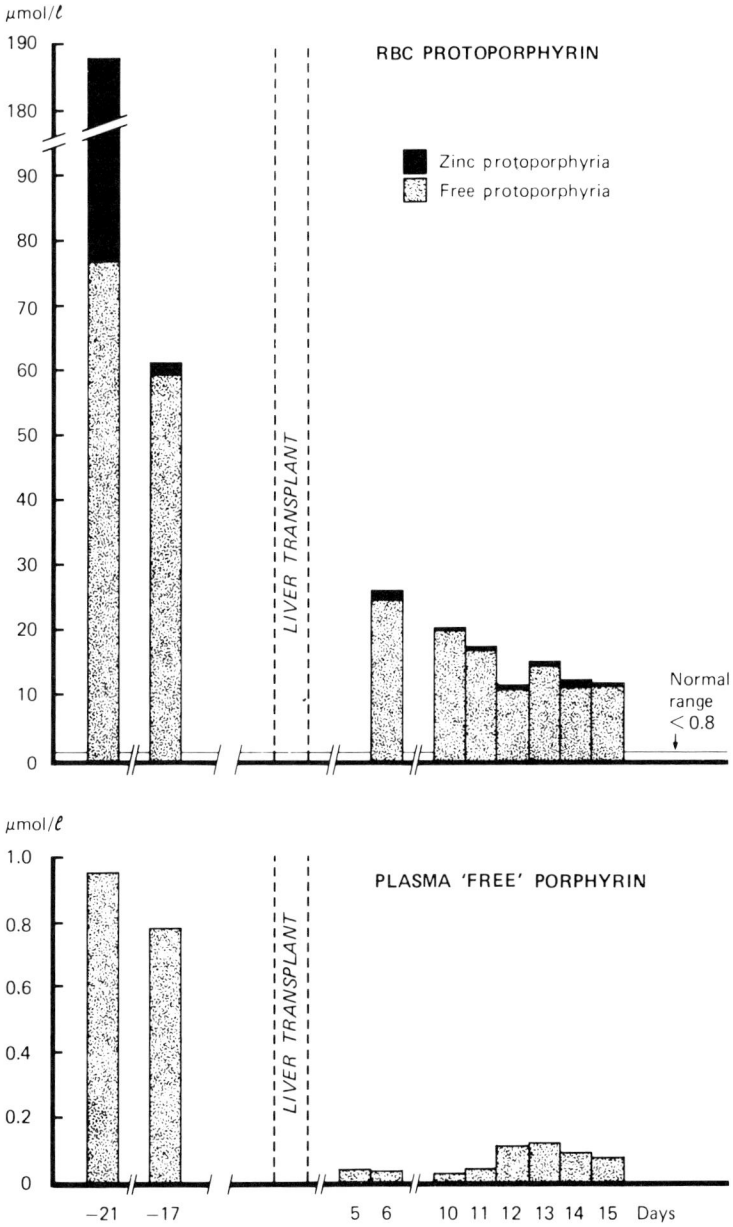

Figure 3. Effects of liver transplantation on porphyrin metabolism in a 13-year-old male with erythropoietic protoporphyria.

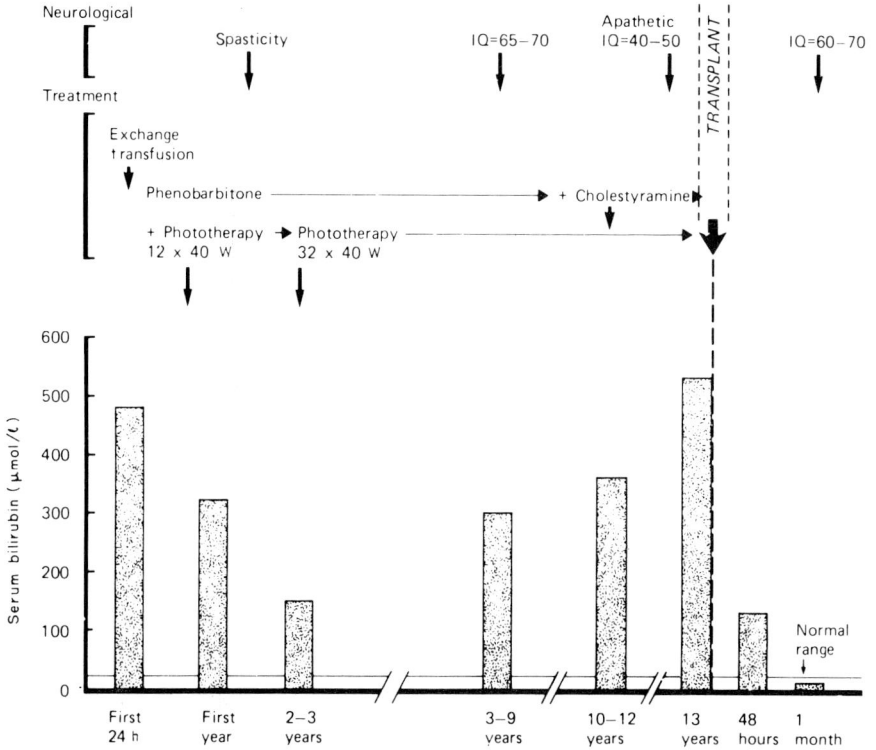

Figure 4. Liver transplantation in a 14-year-old male with Crigler-Najjar syndrome—type 1.

familial hypercholesterolaemia which provided sufficient low-density lipoprotein receptors in the normal donor liver to restore lipid metabolism to normal (Bilheimer et al, 1984; Starzl et al, 1984). Liver transplantation in a 14-year-old boy with type 1 Crigler-Najjar syndrome led to a rapid fall in serum bilirubin levels, although it is too early to say whether or not there will be any mental improvement (Figure 4).

Acute hepatic failure

Although there have been difficulties in using liver transplantation to treat acute hepatic failure (Williams and Gimson, 1984; Van Thiel et al, 1986), it has now become apparent that many centres are having successful results in spite of anticipated problems with bleeding, haemodynamic instability and other end-organ complications. In the Cambridge/King's College Hospital series we now have experience of treating 16 patients with acute liver failure by liver grafting (Table 6). This includes eight patients with fulminant hepatic failure, six with late-onset hepatic failure (with the onset of encephalopathy 8–26 weeks after the onset of symptoms) and two with severe hepatic failure but without encephalopathy. Of these, 13 showed marked early improvement following the transplant and 10 are currently alive.

With regard to timing of the operation, those with fulminant hepatic failure from presumed non-A, non-B hepatitis, idiosyncratic drug reactions, halothane hepatitis and Wilson's disease, in addition to patients with late-onset hepatic failure, have poor prognoses and therefore should be considered early for transplantation. For fulminant hepatic failure secondary to paracetamol overdose, hepatitis A or B infection, the decision is more difficult, as the survival rates with intensive liver care at King's College Hospital are usually between 39 and 67%, depending on which complications are present (Table 7). Transplantation should be carried out before grade IVb encephalopathy and the sequence of advanced cerebral oedema have become established, as in Starzl's series there has been a 50% mortality in this group, partly as a result of irreversible brain damage. In addition the possibility of recurrence of fulminant non-A, non-B hepatitis in the grafted liver has to be considered, as this may account for the otherwise unexplained graft failure 5–6 days post transplantation in two of our cases, and a milder hepatic illness in a third patient at a similar time.

Immunosuppression including Cyclosporin A

In most centres cyclosporin A (CyA) is started immediately after the operation although in our series, because of the drug's nephrotoxicity, we continue to use prednisolone and azathioprine for the first 3–4 days until urine output and electrolytes are satisfactory. Intravenous CyA is then started and the dose of

Table 7. Specific problems of liver grafting in patients with fulminant hepatic failure.

?? Recurrence of NANB viral hepatitis ($n = 9$)		
Fulminant liver failure	2	22.9%
(at 4–9 days)		
Benign viral hepatitis	1	11.1%
Coagulopathy/haemorrhage ($n = 15$)		
DIC syndrome	1	
Severe haemorrhage	2	20.0%
Neurological sequelae ($n = 15$)		
Cortical blindness	1	
(resolving)		13.4%
Bilateral paresis	1	
(resolved)		
Respiratory failure	1	6.7%

azathioprine gradually reduced. When clamping of the T-tube is started and oral intake is satisfactory, usually in the second postoperative week, half the CyA dose is given by mouth. Intravenous administration, however, usually continues for a further 2–3 weeks until the T-tube is fully clamped and the serum bilirubin is less than 100 μmol/l. After the first three months many patients can be maintained on CyA together with low-dose prednisolone; often even this can subsequently be withdrawn.

Work by Starzl's group on the pharmacokinetics of CyA metabolism has shown that when it is taken orally with food after an overnight fast, bile output and hence CyA absorption are increased, resulting in peak and trough drug levels which are approximately twice those seen when the drug is taken alone. A similar enhancement of bioavailability is seen when the T-tube is clamped around the time of CyA administration. Being aware of these factors allows the dose of CyA required to maintain adequate immunosuppressive to be reduced and results in significant financial savings.

The major problem with using CyA after transplantation is its well-established nephrotoxicity (Hamilton et al, 1981; Myers et al, 1984) although this has been shown to be at least partially dose-dependent and reversible on dose reduction (Williams et al, 1985a). In a recent study on 24 patients who had undergone liver graftings and had received CyA for periods of up to $4\frac{1}{2}$ years DTPA scanning and in some cases renal biopsy were used to assess CyA nephrotoxicity. All but one had abnormalities on renal scan with 18 having evidence of reduced renal blood flow. The changes on renal biopsy in six patients showed features of glomerulosclerosis and arteriopathy similar to those seen in ischaemia. These changes may occur because of high blood levels of CyA and may be particularly severe in the early postoperative period when other factors such as hypotension and nephrotoxic antibodies may also be causing renal impairment.

Long-term Rehabilitation and Current Results

Two-thirds of deaths after liver transplantation occur within the first three months; in patients who survive beyond this and who leave hospital, rehabilitation is usually excellent. Many return to school or to full-time work, while of immense satisfaction to the women has been the ability to look after their family and house again. In those dying a year or more after transplantation, the cause of death has been either recurrence of malignant disease or unrelated to the transplant or original disease, such as a myocardial infarction or colonic carcinoma.

As there have been major changes in surgical technique, patient selection and immunosuppressive therapy over the years during which liver transplantation has been performed, it is more relevant to examine current results in different centres than to look back at overall results. In addition it must be remembered that results will depend on the nature and condition of patients selected and this will vary from centre to centre. In the Cambridge/King's College Hospital pro-

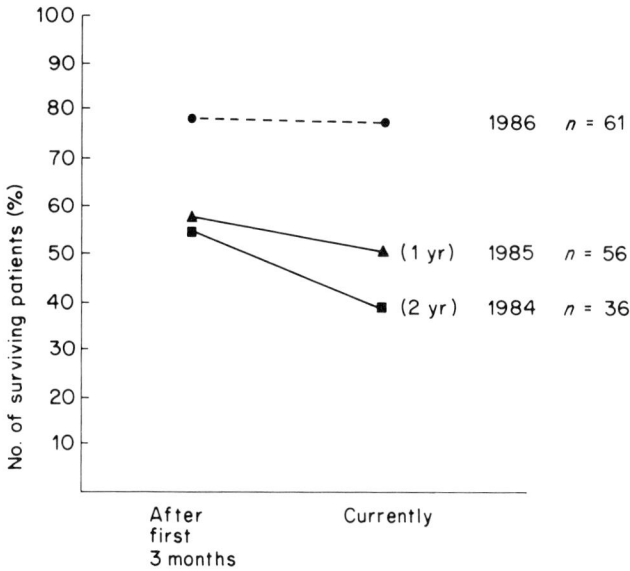

Figure 5. Survival figures for liver-grafted patients in the Cambridge/King's College Hospital series, 1984–26 November 1986.

gramme more patients have had transplants in the last three years than were treated in the preceding 15 years, and the actuarial one-year survival for this recent period is 50%, compared with 28% for the earlier years. It is of further interest that within the last three years, survival figures have continued to improve with fewer deaths in both the initial and later postoperative periods (Figure 5). Although this improvement can in part be explained by an increase in the number of transplants carried out in younger patients who usually have a better survival (Williams et al, 1985b), there has also been a definite improvement in survival of older patients. Of the 47 adult patients undergoing liver grafting in the Cambridge/King's College Hospital series in 1986, 34 are currently alive. In Pittsburgh the latest published actuarial one-year survival for adult transplants is 60% (Van Thiel et al, 1986), with even better figures for children reported previously (Gartner et al, 1984). Similarly in Minneapolis between 1983 and 1985, the actuarial two-year survival was 60%, while in Memphis it was 62% for the same period.

Now that patients can reasonably be offered a liver graft before they are actually in the terminal phase of their disease, immediate survival results will almost certainly continue to improve. When considering survival figures it is also important to take into account the frequency of retransplantation. Patients whose grafts do badly for any reason are best treated by early retransplantation, although such a policy is of course only possible when there is an adequate supply of suitable donor organs. In Starzl's series, around 30% of patients are retransplanted while 5–10% require a third graft, compared with only 10% undergoing retransplantation in our series.

References

Bilheimer DW, Goldstein JL, Grundy SM, Starzl TE and Brown MS (1984) Liver transplantation to provide low-density lipoprotein receptors and lower plasma cholesterol in a child with homozygous familial hypercholesteraemia. *N. Engl. J. Med.* **311**, 1658–64.

Bontempo FA, Lewis JH, Van Thiel DH et al (1985) The relation of preoperative coagulation finding to diagnosis, blood usage and survival in adult liver transplantation. *Transplantation* **39**, 532–6.

Calne RY, Rolles K, Forman JV et al (1984) Veno-arterial bypass in orthotopic liver grafting. *Lancet* **ii**, 1269.

Cuervas-Mons V, Millan I, Gavaler JS, Starzl TE and Van Thiel DH (1986) Prognostic value of preoperatively obtained clinical and laboratory data in predicting survival following orthotopic liver transplantation. *Hepatology* **6**, 922–7.

Fennell RH, Shikes RH and Vierling JN (1983) Relationship of pretransplant hepatobiliary disease to bile duct damage occurring in the liver allograft. *Hepatology* **3**, 84–9.

Gartner JC, Zitelli BJ, Malatack JJ et al (1984) Orthotopic liver transplantation in children: two year experience with 47 patients. *Paediatrics* **74**, 140–5.

Hamilton DV, Calne RY, Evans DB et al (1981) The effect of long-term cyclosporin A on renal function. *Lancet* **i**, 1218–9.

Mittal R, Kowal C, Starzl T et al (1984) Accuracy of computerised tomography in determining hepatic tumour size in patients receiving liver transplantation or resection. *J. Clin. Oncol.* **2**, 637–42.

Myers DB, Ross J, Newton L, Luetscher J and Perlroth M (1984) Cyclosporin-associated chronic nephropathy. *N. Engl. J. Med.* **311**, 699–705.

IHCDC Statement (1984) Liver Transplantation—June 20–23, 1983. *Hepatology* **4**, Supplement.

Neuberger JM, Portmann B, Macdougall B, Calne RY and Williams R (1982) Recurrence of primary biliary cirrhosis after liver transplantation. *N. Engl. J. Med.* **206**, 1–4.

Neuberger JM, Portmann B, Calne RY and Williams R (1984) Recurrence of autoimmune chronic active hepatitis following orthotopic liver grafting. *Transplantation* **37**, 363–5.

Neuberger JM, Altman DG, Christensen E, Tygstrup N and Williams R (1986) Use of a prognostic index in liver transplantation for primary biliary cirrhosis. *Transplantation* **41**, 713–6.

Shaw BW, Martin DJ, Marquez JM et al (1984) Venous bypass in clinical liver transplantation. *Ann. Surg.* **200**, 524–34.

Starzl TE, Bilheimer DW, Bahnson HT et al (1984) Heart-liver transplantation in a patient with familial hypercholesteraemia. *Lancet* **i**, 1382–3.

Van Thiel DH, Udani M, Schade RR, Sanghvi A and Starzl TE (1985) Prognostic value of thyroid hormone levels in patients evaluated for liver transplantation. *Hepatology* **5**, 862–6.

Van Thiel DH, Tarter R, Gavaler JSD, Potanko WM and Schade RR (1986) Liver transplantation in adults. An analysis of costs and benefits at the University of Pittsburgh. *Gastroenterology* **90**, 211–6.

Wall WJ, Duff JH, Ghent CN et al (1985) Liver transplantation: the initial experience of a Canadian centre. *Can. J. Surg.* **28**, 286–9.

Watts RWE, Calne RY, Williams R et al (1985) Primary hyperoxaluria (Type 1): attempted treatment by combined hepatic and renal transplantation. *Q. J. Med.* **57**, 697–703.

Williams R and Gimson AES (1984) An assessment of orthotopic liver transplantation in acute liver failure. *Hepatology* **4**, 22S–24S.

Williams R, Blackburn A, Neuberger J and Calne RY (1985a) Long-term use of cyclosporin in liver grafting. *Q. J. Med.* **57**, 897–905.

Williams R, Calne RY, Rolles K and Polson RJ (1985b) Current results with orthotopic liver grafting in the Cambridge/King's College Hospital series. *Br. Med. J.* **290**, 49–52.

Key Developments in Gastroenterology
Edited by P. R. Salmon
© 1988 John Wiley & Sons Ltd

4

Alcoholic Liver Disease

Sheila Sherlock
Royal Free Hospital School of Medicine, London

In Western countries, the incidence of cirrhosis can be directly related to the quantity of alcohol consumed. In France, between 1941 and 1947, rationing of wine from 5 to 1 litre per week led to an 80% reduction in mortality from cirrhosis (Péquignot and Cyrulnic, 1970). Cirrhosis is increasing and, in the USA, it is the fourth commonest cause of death in white males. In the UK, deaths from cirrhosis have increased by approximately 25% in the last decade. The death rate in different communities correlates quite well with alcohol consumption. The prevalence in various countries depends largely on religious and other customs and on the relation between the cost of alcohol and the weekly wage. In Britain, the relative cost of alcoholic drinks has fallen so that a bottle of spirits is now a third cheaper than in 1965. The lower the cost of alcohol, the lower the socio-economic group affected. Certain occupations are particularly associated with the risks of alcoholism. They include the liquor trade, 'show business' and those on expense accounts or with ready access to duty-free liquor.

During the last ten years, alcoholic liver disease has increased markedly among women (Morgan and Sherlock, 1977; Saunders et al, 1981). They are less likely to be suspected of alcohol abuse. They present at a later stage and are more likely to relapse after treatment.

Each bottle of spirits contains 240 g absolute alcohol. 'Safe' daily consumption is uncertain: 160 g daily used to be the limit, but now 60 g in men, and a mere 20 g in women, may suffice (Péquignot and Cyrulnic, 1970).

Alcoholics with cirrhosis have usually consumed about 190 g of alcohol daily for 10 years, although there are wide individual variations. Alcoholism of short duration may be compensated by a higher daily dose and vice versa.

The liver injury is related not to the type of beverage consumed, but to its alcoholic content. The non-alcoholic constituents of the drink, congeners, are not particularly hepatotoxic. Steady daily imbibers are much more at risk than the spree drinker whose total alcohol intake may be no less. This is partly because the intermittent drinker gives his liver a chance to repair, and partly

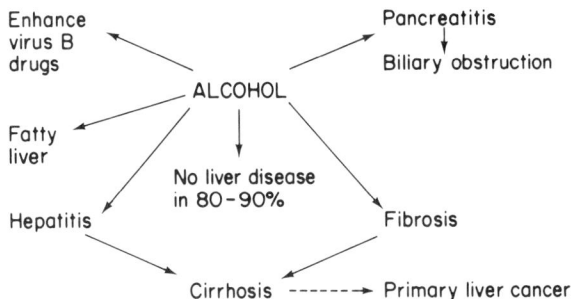

Figure 1. The effects of alcohol abuse on the hepatobiliary
system. Note the 80–90% with no overt liver disease.

because his diet suffers less. Abstinence for at least two days each week is
recommended for everyone and especially those who abuse alcohol.

Not everyone who drinks excessively develops liver damage. In a group of 417
unselected male alcoholics receiving treatment, liver function tests showed severe
liver damage in a quarter, and less liver damage in a half (Lelbach, 1976). The
numerous chronic alcoholics with completely normal livers pose an interesting
problem. There must be genetic influences in determining hepatic susceptibility.
Those that develop alcoholic liver damage are only mildly dependent on alcohol
(Wodak et al, 1983). They escape the florid symptoms of alcohol dependence,
such as withdrawal symptoms, and are at greater risk of developing liver damage
because they are able to maintain a high consumption over many years. Alcohol
has various effects on the hepatobiliary system (Figure 1). It causes fatty liver
(Figure 2). It leads to hepatic cirrhosis. This may be through an intermediary
stage of acute alcoholic hepatitis or simply directly from hepatic fibrosis (Popper
and Lieber, 1980). There is probably a relationship betwen alcohol and primary
liver cancer (Lieber et al, 1986). Chronic alcoholic pancreatitis may be followed
by biliary obstruction and biliary cirrhosis. Finally, alcohol is an enzyme inducer
affecting the metabolism of various drugs. It enhances the effects of hepatitis B
(Villa et al, 1982). The reason why 80–90% of alcoholics have no clinically
obvious liver disease remains unexplained.

Mechanisms of Liver Damage

Relation to alcohol and its metabolites

In Lieber's study (1982), the baboon consuming 50% of total calories as alcohol
in 2–5 years developed cirrhosis. In another study, baboons receiving 70% of
their calories as alcohol with an adequate diet for 30 months failed to show
significant liver damage (Ainley et al, 1984). Evidence for the direct hepatotoxic

ETHANOL

NAD

ADH → HYDROGEN

NADH

Replaces fatty acid as fuel

ACETALDEHYDE
(Toxic)

Ketosis ← Fatty acids

Triglycerides

Acetate

Fatty Liver   Hyperlipidaemia

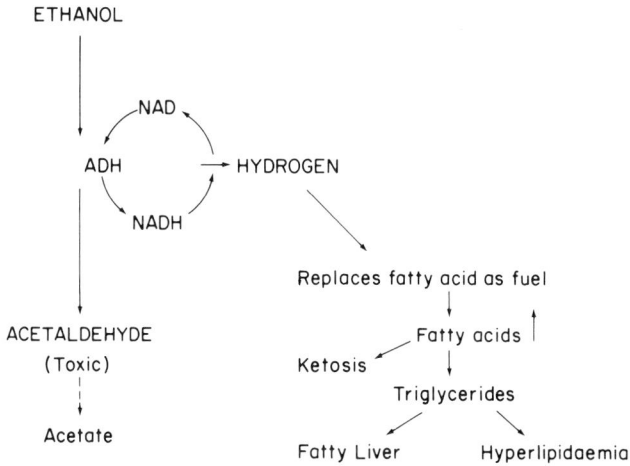

Figure 2. The oxidation of alcohol by the hepatocyte and alcohol dehydrogenase (ADH). The production of acetaldehyde (toxic) is enhanced. The hydrogen produced replaces fatty acid as a fuel so that fatty acids accumulate with consequent ketosis, triglyceridaemia, fatty liver and hyperlipidaemia.

effect of alcohol in man comes from human volunteers, who after 280–560 ml of 86% proof alcohol daily for 8–10 days developed fatty change and EM abnormalities on liver biopsy (Lieber, 1982).

Acetaldehyde is the major product of ethanol oxidation (Figure 2). It is metabolically extremely reactive and toxic. It binds to phospholipids, amino acid residues and sulphydryl groups. It reacts with serotonin, dopamine and noradrenaline, yielding pharmacologically active compounds. It affects the plasma membranes by depolymerising proteins and producing altered surface antigens.

It may inhibit the secretion of newly synthesised glycoprotein and albumin by the hepatocyte. This results in a defect in protein export with retention of water in proportion to the protein (Barasna et al, 1977).

Intracellular redox potential

The marked increase in the NADH:NAD ratio in hepatocytes actively oxidising produces profound metabolic consequences. The altered redox potential has been implicated in the pathogenesis of fatty liver, collagen formation, altered steroid metabolism and impaired gluconeogenesis (Lieber, 1982).

Hypermetabolic state

Chronic alcohol ingestion results in an increased consumption of oxygen. This seems largely to be due to the increased mitochondrial reoxidation of NADH.

The increased oxygen requirement in the liver following chronic alcohol consumption results in a steeper oxygen gradient along the sinusoidal length so that cell necrosis is in zone 3 (centrizonal). It is conceivable that necrosis in this area may be hypoxic in origin (Orrego et al, 1981).

Nutrition

The relation of alcoholic liver damage to nutrition is controversial (Sherlock, 1984). Its role in the perpetuation or initiation of alcoholic liver disease cannot be discounted (Phillips, 1983). It seems likely that both alcohol and nutrition play a part in alcoholic hepatotoxicity, alcohol being the more important. There may be a range of alcohol intake that is tolerated without liver damage under optimal dietary conditions. However, it is also likely that there is a threshold of alcohol toxicity beyond which no protection is afforded by dietary manipulation.

Immunological liver damage

Occasional progression of liver injury despite cessation of alcohol intake has been attributed to immunological mechanisms. Circulating liver membrane antibodies against ethanol-altered rabbit hepatocytes have been detected in patients with alcoholic liver disease (Neuberger et al, 1984).

Acetaldehyde may be concerned. Mallory's alcoholic hyaline has been suggested as a likely neo-antigen (Kanagasundaram et al, 1977). Immunological mechanisms may be concerned in the perpetuation of liver damage in a limited number of alcoholics who show abnormal immunological responses.

Early Recognition of Alcoholic Liver Disease

This depends on a high index of suspicion on the part of the physician. A patient may present with non-specific digestive symptoms such as anorexia, morning nausea with dry retching, diarrhoea, vague right abdominal pain and tenderness or pyrexia.

The patient may seek medical advice because of the effects of alcoholism, such as social disruption, poor work performance, accidents, violent behaviour, fits, tremulousness or depression.

Self-administered screening questionnaires may be useful in detection of alcoholism (Lumeng, 1986).

The diagnosis may be made when hepatomegaly, a raised serum transaminase or macrocytosis are discovered at routine examination—for instance a life insurance check or during investigation of another condition. Physical signs may be non-contributory, although tender hepatomegaly, prominent vascular spiders and associated features of alcoholism may be helpful. The clinical features do not reflect the hepatic histology and biochemical tests of liver function may be normal.

Biochemical tests

Serum transaminase levels are only modestly increased. The relatively low serum aspartate transaminase levels and the high SGOT:SGPT ratio are reflected by changes in the liver activities of these enzymes. Pyridoxal 5-phosphate, the biologically active form of vitamin B_6, is necessary for the activity of both transaminases. In alcoholics, pyridoxal 5-phosphate depletion is partially responsible for the high SGOT:SGPT ratio (Diehl et al, 1984). In alcoholic liver disease, this ratio usually exceeds 2. The mitochondrial isoenzyme of aspartate transaminase (mAST) may be a particularly sensitive index of alcoholic liver disease (Nalpas et al, 1986).

The serum γ-glutamyl transpeptidase (γ-GTP) is a widely used screening test for alcohol abuse. The rise results mainly from hepatic induction of the enzyme, although hepatocellular damage and cholestasis may contribute. There are many false positives due to factors other than alcohol, such as drugs, other diseases and the patient having a value at the upper limit of the normal range.

Serum glutamate dehydrogenase rises with recent alcohol consumption but is not diagnostic of alcoholic hepatitis, nor does it reflect severity of liver damage (Jenkins et al, 1982).

Serum alkaline phosphatase may be markedly increased (greater than four times normal) especially in those with severe cholestasis and alcoholic hepatitis. Serum IgA values may be very high. Serum procollagen type III peptide may be a marker of hepatic fibrogenesis in alcoholic hepatitis and be useful in assessing the progress to cirrhosis (Torres-Salinas et al, 1986).

Various combinations of haematological and biochemical tests have been advocated. Using quadratic, multiple, discriminant analysis of 25 commonly ordered laboratory tests, 100% of non-alcoholics without overt liver disease, 98% of alcoholism treatment programme patients with mild liver involvement, 96% of alcoholics with liver disease and 89% of non-alcoholics with liver disease were correctly classified (Ryback et al, 1982).

Even sensitive biochemical methods may fail to reveal alcoholic liver damage, and liver biopsy must be resorted to in cases of doubt.

Haematological changes

Macrocytosis (MCV greater than 95 μml) is very useful for screening. It is presumably due to a direct effect of alcohol on the bone marrow.

Deficiencies of folate and vitamin B_{12} contribute in the malnourished.

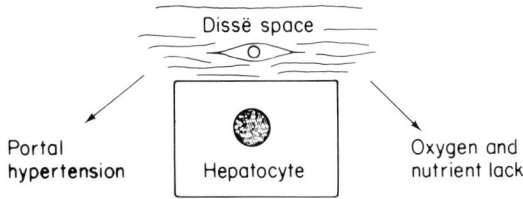

Figure 3. Alcohol leads to fibrosis (perivenular collagen) in
Dissë's space leading to portal hypertension and hepatocyte
deprivation of oxygen and nutrients (Sherlock, 1986).

Liver biopsy

This confirms the presence of liver disease and identifies alcohol abuse as the likely cause. The dangers of the liver damage can be emphasised more forcibly to the patient.

Liver biopsy is important prognostically. Fatty change alone is not nearly so serious as perivenular sclerosis, which is a precursor of cirrhosis (Sørensen et al, 1984). An established cirrhosis can be confirmed.

Diagnostic difficulties may arise when the histological picture of alcoholic liver disease is shown in a patient who denies alcohol abuse. Other causes are Indian childhood cirrhosis, gross obesity, jejunoileal bypass operation, Wilson's disease, diabetes mellitus, prolonged parenteral nutrition and drugs such as perihexiline or amiodarone.

Portal hypertension

Splenomegaly is not prominent. Portal hypertension and gastrointestinal bleeding, however, are frequent at all stages.

The portal hypertension may be related to cirrhosis. Fatty change and centrizonal collagenosis (perivenular sclerosis) leads to a presinusoidal portal hypertension (Goodman and Ishak, 1982). Collagenisation of the space of Dissë decreases sinusoidal diameter, increases resistance to sinusoidal blood flow and raises portal pressure (Orrego et al, 1981) (Figure 3). An increase in hepatocyte volume may also be a factor (Blendis et al, 1982).

Fatty Liver

Mechanism

The fatty change is multifactorial. There is increased delivery of fatty acids to the liver from adipose tissue. Fatty acid synthesis in the liver is increased. Hydrogen replaces fatty acid as a fuel and there is decreased oxidation of hepatic fatty acids (Figure 2). Finally, there is impaired removal of hepatic triglyceride as VLDL particles, due to failure of synthesis of apoprotein.

Hepatic histology

The picture is of macrovesicular fat; occasionally some microvesicular steatosis may also be seen. This is believed to represent fat in transition to large droplets. The macrovesicular fat is present as one or two large globules pushing the nucleus of the hepatocyte to one pole with margination of the cytoplasm (Figure 4). In formol-fixed haematoxylin stained sections, fat appears as punched-out empty vacuoles. It is essential, especially with minor degrees of fatty change, to confirm the presence of fat by the use of a specific stain such as oil-red-O on frozen sections. Connective tissue stains are also essential to determine the existence of zone 3 fibrosis or of cirrhosis.

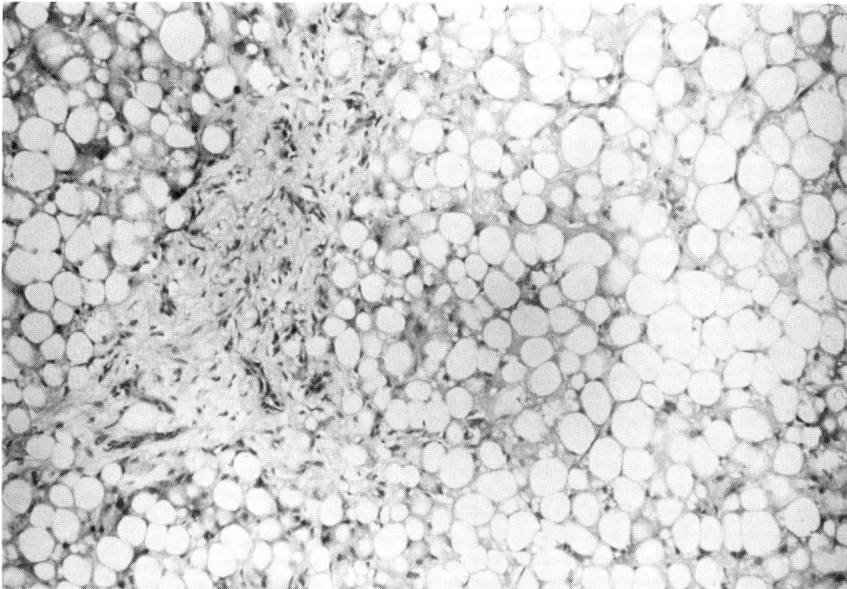

Figure 4. Hepatic histology shows macrovesicular (large droplet) fatty change. The portal tract is expanded and fibrosed suggesting that this patient also suffered from chronic pancreatitis. Stained H & E × 85.

Clinical features

The patients are usually asymptomatic, diagnosis being made when an enlarged, smooth firm liver is discovered. In these patients liver function tests may be normal or the transaminases and alkaline phosphatase slightly increased. If the alcoholic fatty liver is sufficiently severe to merit admission to hospital the patient has usually been drinking heavily for some time and has lost his appetite. There may be nausea and vomiting with periumbilical, epigastric or right upper quadrant pain. Clinically, the fatty liver patient cannot be separated from one with mild alcoholic hepatitis. Needle liver biopsy is essential to diagnose alcoholic hepatitis.

Demonstration of fatty liver

Ultrasound

This shows fat as bright areas of increased echogenicity but of normal attenuation. The sensitivity of the technique is 94% and specificity 84% (Saverymuttu et al, 1986).

CT scanning

This shows the liver with a lower radiological density than normal (Figure 5).

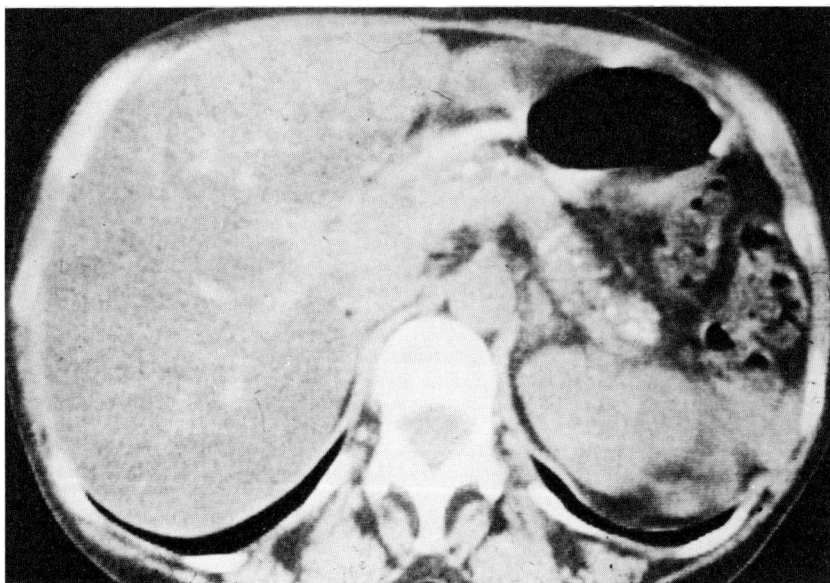

Figure 5. CT scan showing an enlarged fatty liver (density less than that of spleen) with chronic calcific pancreatitis.

Attenuation values are considerably less than those of the spleen and kidneys. The portal vein radicles appear particularly prominent. Monoenergetic CT may be used to assess liver fat content (Bydder et al, 1980). Results agree with chemical and hepatic histological assessment of liver fat. This technique, however, is not generally available.

Prognosis and treatment

Prognosis is good. If the patient is abstinent the fat disappears within about six weeks. However, if the fat is associated with perivenular sclerosis the prognosis is much worse. Treatment consists of stopping alcohol and giving a good balanced diet. No drug is of any proven value.

Alcoholic Hepatitis

Histology

This may occur separately or be combined with an established cirrhosis. Hepatocytes are swollen, and the cytoplasm is granular, firm and often dispersed into fine strands. The nucleus is small and hyperchromatic. Mallory's alcoholic hyaline bodies are seen as intracytoplasmic inclusions within swollen hepatocytes; they usually stain a purplish red with haematoxylin and eosin, but are more readily seen with connective-tissue stains like Masson's trichrome or chromotrope aniline blue. They are found in centrizonal areas and they may persist for as long as six months after alcohol withdrawal. They indicate a more severe hepatitis (Galambos, 1974). Mallory bodies consist of intermediate filaments of varying thickness which are randomly orientated (French, 1981). They are apparently connected to plasma membrane vesicles and the nucleus; they may result from failure of microtubules which is known to lead to intermediate filament increase within the hepatocyte.

The polymorph reaction is related to necrotic and Mallory-containing hepatocytes, polymorphs being arrayed around them in satellite fashion.

Giant mitochondria form globular intracytoplasmic inclusions. They denote milder clinical severity, lower incidence of cirrhosis, fewer complications and longer survival (Chedid et al, 1986).

Pericellular fibrosis is centrizonal. The collagen fibres are perisinusoidal and enclose normal or ballooned hepatocytes. The picture produced is like lattice or chicken wire. Collagenisation of the space of Dissë can be shown by electron microscopy.

Obliteration of the terminal hepatic venules with perivenular fibrosis (phlebosclerosis) is a universal finding (Baptista et al, 1981).

Veno-occlusive lesions and lymphocytic phlebitis have also been described (Goodman and Ishak, 1982), but are much rarer (Burt and MacSween, 1986).

Portal zone changes are inconspicuous with mild to moderate chronic inflammatory infiltrate in the advanced case. Marked portal zone fibrosis suggests a complicating chronic pancreatitis (Morgan et al, 1978b) (Figure 4). The histological patterns form a spectrum from minimal alcoholic hepatitis to an advanced, probably irreversible, picture where necrosis is more extensive and fibrotic scars form (Baptista et al, 1981). Alcoholic hepatitis can be regarded as a precursor of cirrhosis.

Clinical features

The clinical picture is variable from a mild syndrome, resembling fatty liver, through to severe, life-threatening liver decompensation. In the milder form, the symptoms are fatigue, anorexia and weight loss, with a large, tender liver. In the more severe, the patient has usually been drinking particularly heavily. The severe hepatic decompensation may be precipitated by vomiting, diarrhoea, and an intercurrent infection such as pneumonia or an infection of urinary tract, or by prolonged anorexia. Otherwise unexplained pyrexia is usual. The patient may be obese, but some features of malnutrition are present in 90% of patients. The blood pressure is usually low, with a hyperdynamic circulation. Signs of associated vitamin deficiencies, such as beri beri, scurvy or a raw, red tongue, are usual in the malnourished ('skid row') type of alcoholic. The liver is very large, smooth, firm and tender. An arterial bruit may be heard over the liver, causing confusion with the diagnosis of primary liver cancer. The spleen is not palpable unless there is a concomitant cirrhosis. Ascites often develops rapidly.

Diarrhoea with steatorrhoea can be related to decreased biliary excretion of bile salts, to pancreatic insufficiency and to a direct, toxic effect of alcohol on the intestinal mucosa.

Patients with acute fatty liver may die suddenly in shock, attributable to pulmonary fat emboli. Sudden deaths have also been reported in hypoglycaemia.

Gastrointestinal haemorrhage is frequently from a local gastric or duodenal lesion, and is secondary to the general bleeding tendency, rather than related to portal hypertension.

Acute alcoholic hepatitis may be confused with acute virus hepatitis. Helpful diagnostic points are the florid vascular spiders, the very large liver and the leucocytosis. Hepatic biopsy appearances are not specific and there are causes other than alcohol.

Laboratory tests

The serum aspartate transaminase is only mildly increased, usually less than 100 IU/ml. SGOT/SGPT ratio is greater than one. Serum alkaline phosphatase levels are usually increased.

The severity is best correlated with the serum bilirubin and prothrombin time after vitamin K administration (Maddrey et al, 1978). Serum IgA is markedly increased with IgG and IgM raised to a much lesser extent, and serum IgM falls with improvement. The serum albumin level is decreased, increasing as the patient improves. Serum cholesterol levels are usually increased. The serum potassium value is particularly low, largely due to the low dietary protein intake, to diarrhoea and to secondary hyperaldosteronism if fluid retention is present. Albumin-bound serum zinc is decreased, and this is related to a low liver zinc concentration not found in patients with non-alcoholic liver disease. The blood urea and creatinine values increase and these reflect severity. They presage the development of the hepatorenal syndrome.

Alcoholic liver disease is associated with severely decreased hepatic vitamin A levels, when liver injury is moderate (fatty liver) and when blood levels of vitamin A and albumin are still unaffected (Leo et al, 1983). A polymorph leucocytosis of about 15–20 $\times$ 10^9 is found in about a third of patients in proportion to the severity of the alcoholic hepatitis.

Hepatic Cirrhosis

Histology

Classically, cirrhosis of the alcoholic is of a micronodular type. No normal lobular architecture can be identified, and central veins are difficult to find. The amount of fat is variable and acute alcoholic hepatitis may or may not co-exist. With continuing necrosis and replacement fibrosis, the cirrhosis may progress from a micro- to a macronodular pattern, but this is usually accompanied by a reduction in steatosis and, when this end-stage picture is reached, an alcoholic aetiology is difficult to confirm on histological grounds.

Increased hepatic iron can be related to increased iron absorption, the iron content of beverages (especially wines), haemolysis and portacaval shunting. Body iron stores are only moderately increased (Jacobovits et al, 1982) and iron deficiency soon follows multiple venesections.

Established cirrhosis can present without a stage of acute alcoholic hepatitis having been recognised clinically or histologically and the picture can resemble any end-stage liver disease. The points suggesting an alcoholic aetiology include the history of alcohol abuse, which may be forgotten, the hepatomegaly and the associated features of alcoholism. Splenomegaly is a late feature. Liver biopsy findings supporting an alcoholic aetiology include a micronodular cirrhosis, pericentral sclerosis and paucity of hepatic veins. In many instances, however, it is impossible on histological grounds to determine an alcoholic cause (Baptista et al, 1981).

Associated features

The occasional, bilaterally enlarged parotids may be analogous to those seen with other types of malnutrition. Gynaecomastia often appears after treatment and is a frequent complication of spironolactone therapy. The testes atrophy and

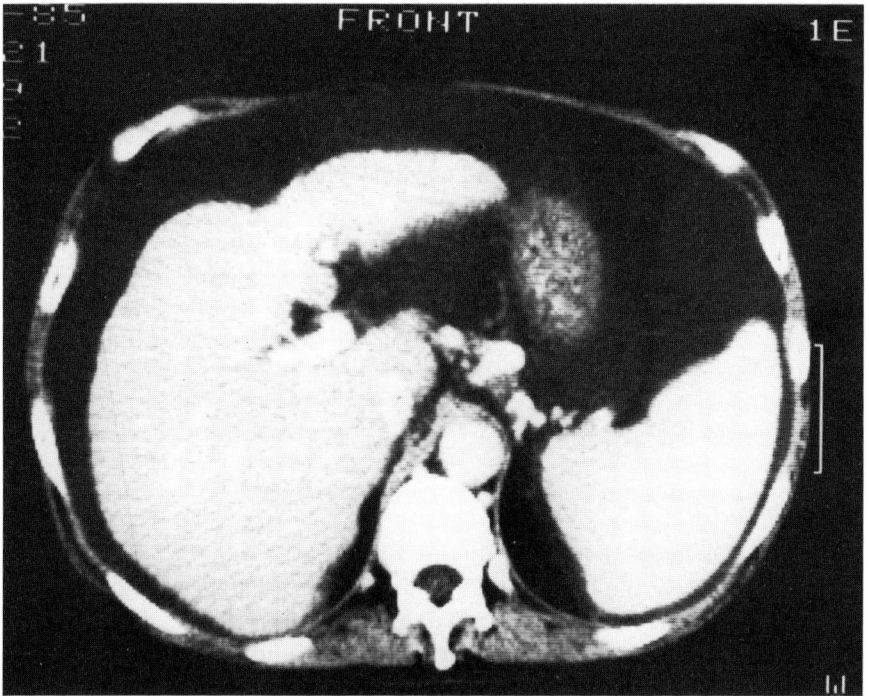

Figure 6. Contrast enhanced CT scan of a cirrhotic liver. Note ascites, irregular liver surface, enlargement of the quadrate lobe of the liver, patent portal vein and splenomegaly.

infertility may be a feature. Muscle mass wastes. Dupuytren's contracture of the palmar fascia is related to the alcoholism and not to the cirrhosis.

Loss of memory and concentration, insomnia, irritability, hallucinations, convulsions, 'rum-fits' and tremor may be the stigmata of alcoholism. These must be distinguished from early hepatic pre-coma. Hepatorenal syndrome seems particularly common in alcoholics.

Renal globular abnormalities, mesangial expansion with deposits of IgA in particular, are frequently found in patients with alcoholic liver disease, showing glomerulonephritis and renal failure. Other constituents of the deposits are Mallory body antigen and complement (Burns et al, 1983).

Scanning procedures

Isotope

In the presence of severe acute alcoholic hepatitis or advanced cirrhosis, isotopes such as technetium are hardly taken up by the liver as the blood shunts past the reticuloendothelial cells.

Ultrasound

This will not detect minimal change, fat or fibrosis. However, in more advanced alcoholic liver disease the liver is diffusely abnormal on ultrasound and the changes correlate with those seen on liver biopsy.

CT scanning

This is well suited to diagnosis of chronic liver disease (Figures 5, 6). The fatty liver shows a lower density than normal. The irregular, nodular liver and its size are shown. The patency of bile ducts and, in the contrast-enhanced scan, main portal and hepatic veins are established. Space occupying lesions, particularly hepatocellular carcinoma, are diagnosed. The presence of ascites is confirmed. Finally, the size and state of spleen, kidneys, pancreas and retroperitoneal portal-venous collaterals are noted.

Prognosis

The prognosis in alcoholics is much better than with other forms of cirrhosis. Everything depends on whether the alcoholic can overcome his addiction. This in turn is related to family support, financial resources and socio-economic state. Overall five-year survival is 50%. If the patient persists in alcoholism this falls to 40%, whereas if they abstain it is 60%.

Of alcoholic patients with non-cirrhotic liver damage 15% will develop cirrhosis during a follow-up period of at least 10 years. Those with liver biopsy appearances of perivenular sclerosis have a worse prognosis than those with fatty change (Sørenson et al, 1984).

Table 1 Minimum daily requirements for an alcoholic (advice to companion) from Sherlock (1984). Reproduced by permission of *The Lancet*.

	Amounts	Remarks
Protein	1 g/kg body weight	Eggs, lean meat, cheese, chicken, liver
Calories	2000	Mixed foods with fruit and vegetables
Vitamins		
A	} One multivitamin tablet	Or one carrot
B complex		Or yeast
C		Or one orange
D		Sunlight
Folate		Good mixed diet
K_1		Good mixed diet

The initial response to treatment is important. Pre-coma, persistent jaundice and azotaemia are bad signs. Such patients are very likely to develop the hepatorenal syndrome. The patient with decompensated cirrhosis improves slowly. Overt jaundice and ascites after three months carry grave prognosis. Even total abstention may not improve the prognosis when portal hypertension is prominent. In this very late, irreversible stage the damage is done and there is no turning back.

Patients with acute alcoholic hepatitis often deteriorate during the first few weeks in hospital. It may take one to six months for resolution, and 20–50% die. Those with markedly prolonged prothrombin time, unresponsive to intramuscular vitamin K, and with a serum bilirubin level greater than 370 IU/l (20 mg/100 dl) have a particularly bad outlook (Maddrey et al, 1978).

Primary liver cancer may develop, particularly in patients who have abstained from alcohol and who have had time to develop a coarsley nodular liver (Lieber et al, 1986).

Treatment

Early recognition

Total abstinence from alcohol is essential. A good diet must be taken and supplementary vitamins, especially B complex, supplied (Table 1) (Sherlock, 1984). Improvement is usually rapid.

After 6–12 months the question of resumption of a modest alcohol intake will arise. The decision is based on the extent of the patient's previous alcohol dependence, his life-style and psychological stability. It also depends on whether the liver biopsy shows centrizonal collagenosis, which is pre-cirrhotic, or simply fatty changes, which may not be. It is possible that all patients who have shown an adverse hepatic reaction to alcohol should abstain forever, but in some instances a small social intake may be allowed. Regular medical check-ups are essential.

Established liver disease

An increased protein intake hastens recovery, but this must be weighed against the possibility of inducing hepatic encephalopathy. Calories, 25–30/kg, and protein, 0.5 g/kg, are given, the latter increasing as soon as possible to 1 g/kg.

In general, nutrients should be given in the form of a normal diet. Nutritional support, whether entered or intravenous, is rarely necessary.

Hepatic failure is marked by a rise in plasma aromatic amino acids together with a fall in branched-chain ones. This has led to the therapeutic use of branched-chain amino acid supplements, particularly in those with hepatic encephalopathy. Results are controversial but little benefit seems to be conferred in terms of encephalopathy or survival (Silk, 1986).

Vitamin B complexes are given in large doses, if necessary parenterally. Potassium chloride supplements are usually required and sometimes additional magnesium, zinc and glucose.

Chlormethiazole (Heminevrin) or chlordiazepoxide (Librium) should be given if the patient has recently been drinking heavily so that delirium tremens may be prevented.

If the diagnosis is in doubt, liver biopsy should be performed as soon as possible, if necessary by the transjugular route. The usual measures for encephalopathy and portal hypertension should be employed. The portal venous pressure may well fall as the alcoholic hepatitis resolves. Surgery should, if possible, be avoided until the maximum benefit has followed medical treatment.

Renal failure is particularly liable to follow hepatocellular failure with ascites in alcoholic patients (hepatorenal syndrome). This has a very bad prognosis.

Corticosteroids improve appetite and consequently augment nutrition. Corticosteroids would also inhibit the cellular immune responses to autologous and homologous liver antigens found in acute alcoholic hepatitis, but the results of therapy have been extremely conflicting. They seem to depend on the type of patient being treated, on the severity of the alcoholic hepatitis and on various other associated features such as the presence or absence of cirrhosis, encephalopathy or renal failure. There seems to be little effect in the mild and moderate case (Depew et al, 1980). However, methyl prednisolone may result in improved short-term survival in patients with severe alcoholic hepatitis (Maddrey et al, 1986).

Testosterone or anabolic-androgenic steroids have been suggested for alcoholic hepatitis and cirrhosis (Maddrey, 1986). In one study, oxandrolone given long term (the patients had to survive 30 days) to those with moderately severe disease decreased mortality (Mendenhall et al, 1984). In a multicentre trial from Denmark, oral testosterone apparently increased mortality (Copenhagen Study Group for Liver Diseases, 1986). In experimental animals, chronic feeding of alcohol leads to hypermetabolic state with an increased rate of oxygen consumption by the liver. This is abolished by pretreatment with propyl thiouracil. The drug has been used short term in patients with active alcoholic liver disease and the rapidity of improvement was enhanced (Orrego et al, 1981). A further double-blind controlled trial of propyl thiouracil in severe alcoholic hepatitis showed no effect on survival or in the frequency or incidence of complications (Halle et al, 1982).

Colchicine inhibits microtubule-mediated transcellular movement of collagen. In a study of 43 cirrhotic patients, of whom 23 received colchicine for at least 48 months as part of a double-blind trial, a significant decrease in liver fibrosis was observed in serial biopsies. Marked clinical improvement occurred, and serum albumin was maintained (Kershenobich et al, 1979). Extension and confirmation of these results is awaited.

Cholestatic Syndromes

The foamy fat syndrome

Occasionally, the patient may present with deep jaundice, hepatomegaly and an increase in serum alkaline phosphatase, transaminase and cholesterol (Morgan et al, 1978a). Functional renal failure is usual. This is usually the first episode of decompensation.

Liver biopsy shows massive accumulation of microvesicular fat with cholestasis in centrizonal areas (Figure 7). Inflammation is inconspicuous and there is little or no Mallory's hyaline. Electron microscopy shows extensive disorganisation of the organelles in affected hepatocytes. The condition has been termed alcoholic foamy degeneration (Uchida et al, 1983). Prognosis is very variable.

Secondary to alcoholic pancreatitis

Cholestasis may be due to compression of the intrapancreatic portion of the common bile duct by chronic alcoholic pancreatitis. Liver biopsy in these patients

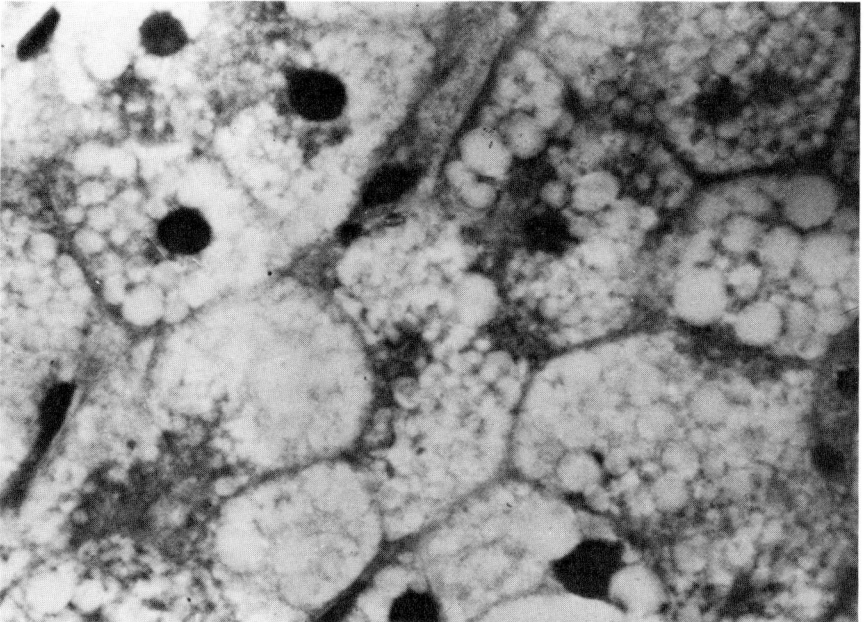

Figure 7. Alcoholic foamy fat syndrome. Note hepatocytes show a foamy appearance due to microvesicular fat. The nucleus is central.

usually shows marked portal zone fibrosis (Morgan et al, 1978) (Figure 4). Endoscopic retrograde cholangiopancreatography (ERCP) confirms the diagnosis. Indeed, bile duct stenosis is very frequent in patients with chronic pancreatitis. It should be suspected in any patient with chronic pancreatitis who shows a serum alkaline phosphatase value exceeding twice normal for more than one month.

Relationship of alcoholic liver disease to hepatitis B

Markers of past or current hepatitis B are more common in patients with alcoholic liver disease than in the general population. There is, however, considerable doubt as to which is the cart and which is the horse, for when liver biopsies are performed the underlying changes are not those of alcoholism, suggesting that hepatitis B or another aetiological agent is the primary event. Alcohol may enhance the liver damage caused by hepatitis B and carriers should be advised to abstain from alcohol or take very small amounts (Villa et al, 1982).

Alcohol as an enzyme inducer

Alcohol ingestion considerably enhances paracetamol toxicity, so that as little as 4–8 g can cause serious liver damage (Sherlock, 1986) (Figure 8). This is apparently because alcohol induces a distinct liver cytochrome, P-450 3a, which is important in

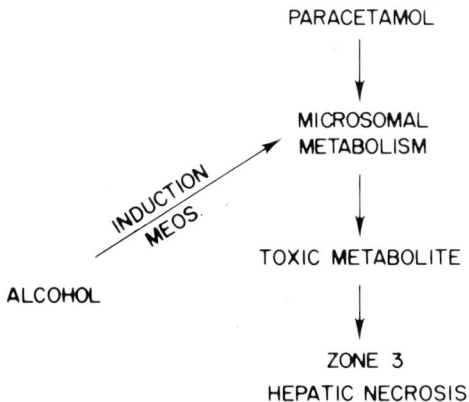

Figure 8. Alcohol, as an enzyme-inducing agent, increases the production of toxic metabolites of paracetamol so potentiating hepatic necrosis (Sherlock, 1986).

generating toxic metabolities. P-450 3a is also concerned in oxygenation of nitro-samines at the alpha carbon. Theoretically, this could increase the risk of cancer in alcoholics (Lieber et al, 1986).

References

Ainley C, Senapati A, Brown IMH et al (1984) Is alcohol hepatotoxic in the baboon? *J. Hepatol.* (Suppl.) **1**, 52.

Baptista A, De Groote J, Bianchi L et al (1981) Alcoholic liver disease: morphological manifestations. *Lancet* **i**, 707–11.

Baraona E, Leo MA, Borowsky SA and Lieber C (1977) Pathogenesis of alcohol-induced accumulation of protein in the liver. *J. Clin. Invest.* **60**, 546–54.

Blendis LM, Orrego H, Crossley IR et al (1982) The role of hepatocyte enlargement in hepatic pressure in cirrhotic and non-cirrhotic alcoholic liver disease. *Hepatology* **2**, 539–46.

Burns J, D'Ardenne AJ, Morton JA et al (1983) Immune complex nephritis in alcoholic cirrhosis: detection of Mallory body antigen in complexes by means of monoclonal antibodies to Mallory bodies. *J. Clin. Path.* **36**, 751–9.

Burt AD and MacSween RNM (1986) Hepatic vein lesions in alcoholic liver disease: retrospective biopsy and necropsy study. *J. Clin. Path.* **39**, 63–7.

Bydder G, Kreel L, Chapman RWG et al (1980) Accuracy of computed tomography in diagnosis of fatty liver. *Br. Med. J.* **281**, 1042–3.

Chedid A, Mendenhall CL, Tosch T et al (1986) Significance of megamitochondria in alcoholic liver disease. *Gastroenterology* **190**, 858–64.

Copenhagen Study Group for Liver Disease (1986) Testosterone treatment of men with alcoholic cirrhosis: a double-blind study. *Hepatology* **6**, 807–13.

Depew W, Boyer T, Omato M, Redeker A and Reynolds T (1980) Double-blind controlled trial of prednisolone therapy in patients with severe acute alcoholic hepatitis and spontaneous encephalopathy. *Gastroenterology* **78**, 524–9.

Diehl AM, Potter J, Boitnott J et al (1984) Relationships between pyridoxal 5-phosphate deficiency and aminotransferase levels in alcoholic hepatitis. *Gastroenterology* **86**, 632–6.

French SW (1981) The Mallory body: structure, composition and pathogenesis. *Hepatology* **1**, 76–83.

Galambos JT (1974) Alcoholic hepatitis. In Schaffner F, Sherlock S and Leevy CM (eds) *Liver Diseases,* pp 255–67. New York: Intercontinental Medical Book Corporation.

Goodman ZD and Ishak KG (1982) Occlusive venous lesions in alcoholic liver disease. *Gastroenterology* **83**, 786–96.

Halle P, Pare P, Kaptein E et al (1982) Double-blind, controlled trial of propylthiouracil in patients with severe acute alcoholic hepatitis. *Gastroenterology* **82**, 925–31.

Jakobovits AW, Morgan MY and Sherlock S (1982) Hepatic siderosis in alcoholics. *Lancet* **i**, 628–9.

Jenkins WJ, Rosalki SB, Foo Y et al (1982) Serum glutamate dehydrogenase is not a reliable marker of liver cell necrosis in alcoholics. *J. Clin. Path.* **35**, 207–10.

Kanagasundaram N, Kakumu S, Chen T et al (1977) Alcoholic hyaline antigen (AHAg) and antibody (AHAb) in alcoholic hepatitis. *Gastroenterology* **73**, 1368–72.

Kershenobich D, Dietrichson O, Loud FB et al (1979) Zinc depletion in alcoholic liver disease. *Scand. J. Gastroenterol.* **15**, 363–7.

Lelbach WK (1976) Epidemiology of alcoholic liver disease. In Popper H and Shaffner F (eds) *Progress in Liver Disease, vol. 5,* pp 494–515. New York: Grune & Stratton.

Leo MA and Lieber CS (1982) Hepatic vitamin A depletion in alcoholic liver injury. *N. Engl. J. Med.* **307**, 597–601.

Leo MA, Sato M and Lieber CS (1983) Effect of hepatic vitamin A depletion on the liver in humans and rats. *Gastroenterology* **84**, 562–72.

Lieber CS (1982) *Medical Disorders of Alcoholism. Pathogenesis and Treatment.* Philadelphia: Saunders.

Lieber CS, Garro A, Leo MA, Mak KM and Worner T (1986) Alcohol and Cancer. *Hepatology* **6**, 1005–19.

Lumeng L (1986) New diagnostic markers for alcohol abuse. *Hepatology* **6**, 742–5.

Maddrey WC (1986) Is therapy with testosterone or anabolic-androgenic steroids useful in the treatment of alcoholic liver disease? *Hepatology* **6**, 1033–35.

Maddrey WC, Carithers RL Jr, Herlong HE et al (1986) Prednisolone therapy in patients with severe alcoholic hepatitis: results of a multicenter trial. *Hepatology* **6** (abstract).

Mendenhall CL, Anderson S, Garcia-Pont P et al (1984) VA cooperative study on alcoholic hepatitis. 1. Acute and long-term survival in patients treated with oxandrolone and prednisolone. *N. Engl. J. Med.* **311**, 1464–70.

Morgan MY and Sherlock S (1977) Sex-related differences among 100 patients with alcoholic liver disease. *Br. Med. J.* **1**, 939–41.

Morgan MY, Sherlock S and Scheuer PJ (1978a) Acute cholestasis, hepatic failure and fatty liver in the alcoholic. *Scand. J. Gastroenterol* **13**, 299–303.

Morgan MY, Sherlock S and Scheuer PJ (1978b) Portal zone fibrosis in the livers of alcoholic patients. *Gut* **19**, 1015–21.

Nalpas O, Charpin, S, Lacou RB and Berthelot P (1986) Serum mitochondrial aspartate aminotransferase as a marker of chronic alcoholism: diagnostic value and interpretation in a Liver Unit. *Hepatology* **6**, 608–14.

Neuberger J, Crossley IR, Saunders JB et al (1984) Antibodies to alcohol-altered liver cell determinants in patients with alcoholic liver disease. *Gut* **25**, 300–8.

Orrego H, Medline A, Blendis LM, Rankin JG and Kreaden DA (1979) Collagenisation of the Dissë space in alcoholic liver disease. *Gut* **20**, 673–9.

Orrego H, Israel Y and Blendis LM (1981) Alcoholic liver disease: information in search of knowledge? *Hepatology* **1**, 267–83.

Orrego H, Israel Y, Blake JE et al (1983) Assessment of prognostic factors in alcoholic liver disease: toward a global quantitative expression of severity. *Hepatology* **3**, 896–912.

Péquignot G and Cyrulnik F (1970) Chronic disease due to overconsumption of alcoholic drinks (excepting neuropsychiatric change). In *International Encyclopaedia of Pharmacology and Therapeutics*, vol. 11, chap. 14, pp 375–412. Oxford: Pergamon Press.

Phillips GB (1983) Acute hepatic insufficiency of the alcoholic—revisited. *Am. J. Med.* **75**, 1–3.

Popper H and Lieber CS (1980) Histogenesis of alcoholic fibrosis and cirrhosis in the baboon. *Am. J. Pathol.* **98**, 695–716.

Ryback RS, Eckardt MJ, Felsher B and Rawlings RR (1982) Biochemical and hematologic correlates of alcoholism and liver disease. *J. A. M. A.* **248**, 2261–5.

Saunders JB, Davis M and Williams R (1981) Do women develop alcoholic liver disease more readily than men? *Br. Med. J.* **282**, 1140–3.

Saverymuttu SH, Joseph AEA and Maxwell JD (1986) Ultrasound scanning in the detection of hepatic fibrosis and steatosis. *Br. Med. J.* **292**, 13–15.

Sherlock S (1984) Nutrition and the alcoholic. *Lancet* i, 436–40.

Sherlock S (1986) The spectrum of hepatotoxicity due to drugs. *Lancet* ii, 440–4.

Silk DBA (1986) Branched chain amino acids in liver disease: fact or fantasy? *Gut* **27**, (S1) 103–10.

Sørensen TIA, Orholm M, Bentsen KD et al (1984) Prospective evaluation of alcohol abuse and alcoholic liver injury in men as predictors of development of cirrhosis. *Lancet* **ii**, 241–5.

Torres-Salinas M, Pares A, Caballeria J et al (1986) Serum procollagen type 111 peptide as a marker of hepatic fibrogenesis in alcoholic hepatitis. *Gastroenterology* **90**, 1241–6.

Uohida T, Kao H, Quispe-Sjogren M et al (1983) Alcoholic foamy degeneration—a pattern of acute alcoholic injury of the liver. *Gastroenterology* **84**, 683–92.

Villa E, Rubbiani L, Barchi T et al (1982) Susceptibility of chronic symptomless HbsAg carriers to ethanol-induced hepatic damage. *Lancet* **ii**, 1243–4.

Wodak AD, Saunders JB, Ewusi-Mensah I et al (1983) Severity of alcohol dependence in patients with alcoholic liver disease. *Br. Med. J.* **287**, 1420–4.

Key Developments in Gastroenterology
Edited by P. R. Salmon
© 1988 John Wiley & Sons Ltd

5

Severe Ulcerative Colitis

D. P. Jewell
Radcliffe Infirmary and University of Oxford, Oxford

Severe attacks of ulcerative colitis are defined as the passage of more than six loose stools daily with blood together with evidence of systematic disturbance, namely fever, tachycardia, anaemia, a tender colon or hypoalbuminaemia (Truelove and Witts, 1955). Before the introduction of corticosteroid drugs, mortality of these severe attacks was in excess of 35% but should now be less than 5%, including operative mortality. Unfortunately this is not universally true and high mortality rates still exist (Ritchie, 1974; Buckell and Lennard-Jones, 1979) although with increasing numbers of trained gastroenterologists in district general hospitals there is some evidence that mortality can be similar to that obtained in specialist centres. To achieve a successful outcome, the severity of the attack must be realised, signs indicating a poor prognosis must be appreciated, aggressive medical therapy should be employed and urgent surgery should not be delayed.

Possible Factors Influencing Mortality

Assessment of severity

The definition of a severe attack is straightforward but many patients who fit the definition given above look well. In these circumstances, the physician can be misled into treating the disease less aggressively. Anorexia, nausea or abdominal pain are worrying symptoms and a tender colon or greatly reduced bowel sounds indicate severe disease. A persistent tachycardia should also alert the physician even though the patient is otherwise well apart from the diarrhoea. This initial assessment of disease severity is greatly helped by documenting those factors which indicate a poor prognosis. In addition, it must be remembered that vital signs such as fever and signs of peritoneal reaction may be suppressed by corticosteroids.

Prognostic factors

Lennard-Jones and his colleagues (1975) have identified by multivariate analysis four clinical features that indicate a poor outlook. Thus, within the first 24 hours of hospital admission, a fever, tachycardia or severe diarrhoea put that patient in the high-risk group for urgent therapy. Likewise, serum albumin concentration of less than 30 g/l within the first four days also predicts that the patient is likely to fail on medical therapy. The actual risk weighting of each of these is given in Table 1. Another useful sign of a poor prognosis is the presence of 'mucosal islands' on the plain abdominal radiograph.

Table 1 The proportion of patients failing to respond to medical therapy in relation to clinical features.

		% failure
In first 24 hours		
Maximum temperature	38°C	56
Maximum pulse rate	> 100/min	36
Bowel frequency	> 9/day	33
	> 12/day	55
Within first four days		
Serum albumin	30 g/l	42

From Lennard-Jones et al (1972).

Corticosteroid dose

Patients are still referred with severe disease 'unresponsive to medical therapy' when that therapy consisted only of sulphasalazine with perhaps topical corticosteroid therapy in addition. Nevertheless, it has been clearly shown that corticosteroids are superior to sulphasalazine for the treatment of active disease (Truelove et al, 1962) and that the therapeutic benefit of corticosteroids is dose dependent (Baron et al, 1962). Thus for patients with mild attacks (less than five stools daily with no systemic disturbance), 20 mg prednisolone should be given daily by mouth with a steroid retention enema or foam preparation, and treatment should combine for at least four weeks before tailing off the oral steroid. For patients with moderately severe attacks (more than five stools daily but still without systemic disturbance), the initial dose of prednisolone should be 40 mg daily reducing to 20 mg over a two-week period and then continuing as for a mild attack. Using such dose regimens, most patients will go into remission and in only a few will the disease progress into a severe attack. When a patient presents with a severe attack, he should be admitted to hospital and treated more aggressively with higher doses of corticosteroids.

Timing of urgent surgery

There is no doubt that surgical mortality is increased if surgery is delayed to the point where the patient becomes malnourished and grossly hypercortocoid. Infection and poor wound healing are then liable to be major problems. Hence the timing of urgent surgery is fairly critical and an experienced surgeon should see all patients with severe attacks of ulcerative colitis in consultation with the physicians. Any patient deteriorating during the first few days of intensive medical therapy should come to surgery and, in Oxford, urgent colectomy is also advised if substantial improvement has not occurred by the end of the first week of therapy (Truelove and Jewell, 1974). Experience has shown that most patients who only make a partial response (i.e., watery diarrhoea with blood in excess of three times daily, persistent tachycardia or a low-grade fever) do not respond to continued medical treatment and ultimately come to surgery.

Management of a Severe Attack

Once the patient is admitted, deficiencies of blood, fluid and electrolytes should be remedied immediately. If the patient is obviously malnourished, total parenteral nutrition should be instituted. Plain abdominal radiographs are mandatory. Stool samples must be sent for culture and to exclude the presence of *Clostridium difficile* toxin. Amoebae must also be excluded. Sigmoidoscopy with rectal biopsy should be performed. However, treatment for ulcerative colitis should begin immediately. Relapses of colitis are only rarely caused by a specific organism (e.g. *Salmonella, Campylobacter*) although it may be impossible to differentiate a first attack of ulcerative colitis from an infective colitis. Rapidity of onset, severe abdominal pain and a history of associated cases, are strongly suggestive of infection but are by no means absolute. In fact, provided amoebiasis can be excluded, corticosteroids are not contraindicated and should be given. In Oxford, patients are given nil by mouth except water; all fluids, electrolytes and corticosteroids are given intravenously (Table 2). Methyl prednisolone or hydrocortisone can be used. In addition, hydrocortisone is given by

Table 2   Intravenous regimen for the treatment of severe ulcerative colitis.

Each 24 hours
Three litres of fluids (including calories)
Potassium
Parenterovite (when indicated)
Methyl prednisolone 64 mg in divided doses

or

Hydrocortisone hemisuccinate, 400 mg in divided doses
Hydrocortisone hemisuccinate 100 mg b.d. by rectal infusion

rectal infusion twice daily in a volume of about 100 ml. It is customary to drip the hydrocortisone in over 15–30 minutes with the patient lying on the left side. The foot of the bed can be elevated if necessary. The advantage of this method is that the enema is usually retained. If a standard retention enema is used, the severely inflamed rectum is unable to hold a sudden bolus and immediately rejects it. This regimen of treatment should continue for 5–7 days. During that time, pulse, temperature and blood pressure will be monitored but, in addition, it is useful to check abdominal girth on a daily basis and to note the presence of bowel sounds. All patients should have repeated abdominal X-rays and these should certainly be done daily for those patients showing the signs of a poor prognosis listed in Table 1. Additional films should be obtained immediately if there is an unexplained rise in pulse or loss of bowel sounds—these are often the only signs to indicate a perforation or an acute dilation of the colon.

Using this procedure for managing severe attacks, 70–75% will go into remission (Truelove and Jewell, 1972; Truelove et al, 1978). Substantial improvement is seen by the end of the first week of treatment such that patients feel well, they are passing no more than one or two motions without blood and the stool is beginning to form. Patients should then be given a light diet, oral prednisolone (40–60 mg daily) and sulphasalazine. If improvement is maintained, they are allowed home by about the tenth day and managed as previously described for a moderate attack.

For patients who do not show considerable improvement during intravenous treatment, urgent colectomy should be advised. Some patients will have shown a partial response and will naturally be reluctant to submit to surgery. In these, it is worth letting them go into oral therapy and to start eating. A few will continue to improve and will eventually go into remission but most will experience an increase in diarrhoea and bleeding, the pulse may rise and fever may recur. Under these circumstances, there should be no delay in proceeding to surgery.

Although this regimen of management has proved to be an effective form of treating severe ulcerative colitis, several questions arise which should be considered.

1. Is bowel rest necessary?

The most severely ill patients are anorectic and nauseated. Thus, they are taking little by mouth and, in any case, may need an intravenous line for electrolytes, fluid and blood replacement. However, whether bowel rest plays a useful role in the management of the attack is not proven. In fact, the evidence so far suggests that it is unnecessary. One study from Leeds randomised patients to receive either intravenous alimentation and bowel rest or a normal diet (Dickinson et al, 1980). Both groups received prednisolone by mouth. No benefit was seen in favour of bowel rest. A similar conclusion was reached in another study which treated severe ulcerative colitis patients with intravenous corticosteroids but then randomised them to intravenous nutrition with bowel rest or an oral diet (McIntyre et al, 1986). Bowel rest did not appear to affect the remission rate or the surgical rate.

Therefore, although the use of bowel rest and intravenous therapy is a convenient and effective form of therapy it is not possible to conclude that bowel rest per se is beneficial.

2. Is there a role for antibiotics?

The earlier retrospective studies from Oxford used intravenous tetracycline during the period of intravenous therapy although it was recognised that its use was purely empirical (Truelove and Jewell, 1974; Truelove et al 1978). Recently two trials of antibiotic therapy for severe attacks of ulcerative colitis have been reported. Chapman et al (1986) treated 39 patients with the intravenous regimen and randomised them to have either intravenous metronidazole or a dummy preparation. Both groups did equally well and no benefit for metronidazole could be seen. Furthermore, the response rates and the surgical rate were virtually identical to the two previous studies which employed tetracycline, suggesting that tetracycline was also of little benefit.

The other controlled trial of antibiotics for severe disease compared oral vancomycin with placebo (Dickinson et al, 1985). Forty patients were admitted to the study, of whom 33 had ulcerative colitis and 7 had Crohn's disease. All had oral prednisolone. No significant difference emerged in favour of vancomycin although fewer patients receiving this antibiotic came to surgery than those having placebo. No evidence of clostridial infection was found.

Thus there is no evidence that antibiotics have a role in the treatment of severe ulcerative colitis.

3. When should barium radiology or colonoscopy be performed?

For patients who are being treated for a severe relapse of established disease, the diagnosis is seldom in doubt, so that a barium enema or colonoscopy are not required in the acute stage. If they are required to determine the extent of disease or to be sure the patient does not have Crohn's disease, they should be delayed until remission has been achieved.

The situation is more difficult in patients presenting in their first attack when the diagnosis may not be clear. Nevertheless, it is best to avoid these diagnostic procedures and it is usually possible to do so given the history, the appearances of the bowel on a plain abdominal X-ray, the sigmoidoscopy appearances and the results of stool culture and rectal biopsy. If there is still diagnostic difficulty which is affecting management, then an 'instant enema' can be performed. In this procedure, the colon is not prepared, balloon catheters are not used, the barium is run into the colon at low pressure and is immediately stopped if pain develops. Double-contrast studies with air insertion and the use of relaxants (e.g. buscopan or glucagon) are absolutely forbidden in severe colitis. Likewise, colonoscopy should not be performed for fear of causing an acute dilation or even a perforation.

4. How should complications be managed?

Acute dilatation of the colon is the most common of the local complications, occurring in about 5% of patients with severe attacks. The diagnosis is made on a plain abdominal X-ray which will show a transverse colon greater than 5.5 cm in diameter. Patients should be treated with intravenous steroids together with fluid and electrolyte replacement. Patients frequently have a metabolic alkalosis which should be corrected (Torsoli, 1981). Many patients will improve on this treatment and ultimately go into remission. However, if there is deterioration in the patient's condition or there is no obvious improvement in 24 hours, urgent colectomy should be performed.

Perforation is a rare but highly dangerous complication. It usually occurs in first attacks and is a definite indication for immediate surgery once fluid and electrolyte balance has been corrected. The patient will also require intravenous antibiotics as well as corticosteroids.

Massive haemorrhage is also a rare complication. Blood transfusion should begin as soon as possible and if bleeding is severe, a central venous pressure line is useful to monitor the patient's haemodynamic state. Intensive medical therapy should begin as already described, but urgent colectomy will be required if bleeding does not stop within six hours or so.

5. Which operation?

Until recently, the operation of choice was a one-stage proctocolectomy even for the most severely ill patients. With an experienced surgeon, the mortality of this operation is very low (<5%). This operation should still be performed for anyone over the age of 50 and for those younger patients who are not judged suitable for the formation of a pelvic, ileoanal pouch. The factors which determine unsuitability include poor anal tone, low intelligence and a brittle psychological make-up.

Nevertheless, the formation of an ileoanal pouch is an alternative to procto-colectomy for the younger patient. In the acute stage, it is preferable to remove the colon but to leave the rectum in situ, bringing it out on to the abdominal wall as a mucous fistula. The whole colon is then available for histological study. If ulcerative colitis is confirmed, the second operation is performed a few months later at which a rectal mucosectomy is performed followed by the fashioning of the pouch.

6. How can treatment be improved?

Even though the overall mortality of a severe attack of ulcerative colitis is now low, there is still a 20–25% chance of a patient requiring urgent colectomy. To be able to reduce this surgical rate would represent a major advance in management. Unfortunately there is little evidence of this happening in the near future, although the use of higher doses of corticosteroids or of immuno-suppressive agents might be worth exploring.

Evidence that ACTH might be more effective than corticosteroids has been conflicting (Jewell and Baker, 1986) although ACTH gel intramuscularly appeared to be significantly better than oral cortisone acetate in the early studies (Truelove and Witts, 1959). More recently, Meyers et al (1983) have suggested that ACTH intravenously is more effective than intravenous hydrocortisone for patients presenting with a severe attack who have not been previously treated with corticosteroids. Conversely, those who had been having oral corticosteroid therapy seemed to gain most benefit from hydrocortisone. However, the differences between the treatment groups are small and any possible benefit of ACTH seems marginal. Pulse therapy with high-dose methyl prednisolone similar to that used following organ transplantation has not been formally tested in ulcerative colitis. However, anecdotal experience in Oxford has not been encouraging.

The immunosuppressive drug most used for the treatment of ulcerative colitis is azathioprine. However, if it does have a role it is as a maintenance agent or as a steroid-sparing agent and it is of no use for active disease (Jewell and Truelove, 1974; Kirk and Lennard-Jones, 1982). This is because, whatever the exact mode of action, any therapeutic benefit is not seen until two or three months of treatment have elapsed. A much more rapidly acting immunosuppressive drug is cyclosporin A which inhibits the release of cytokines from macrophages and lymphocytes. We have recently studied 12 patients with severe attacks of ulcerative colitis. All patients were given intravenous corticosteroids as de-scribed above but they also had cyclosporin by mouth. The initial dose was high (15 mg/kg/day) but was slowly tapered off over six weeks. No obvious benefit was seen with six of the 12 patients requiring urgent surgery (K Baker and D P Jewell, unpublished observations).

Conclusions

Mortality of severe attacks of ulcerative colitis has fallen dramatically during the last two decades and should now be less than 5%. This has been brought about by the better recognition of severe disease in a patient who looks well, by aggressive treatment of mild or moderate attacks and by the standardisation of a protocol for the management of these severe attacks. Close cooperation with an experienced surgeon ensures that surgery is timed correctly for the patient who is not responding to medical therapy and also ensures that surgical mortality is rare.

The challenge for the future is to improve medical therapy and so reduce the risk of urgent colectomy.

References

Baron JH, Connell AM, Kanaghinis TG, Lennard-Jones JE and Jones FA (1962) Outpatient treatment of ulcerative colitis: Comparison between three doses of oral prednisolone. *Br. Med. J.* **2**, 441–3.

Buckell NA and Lennard-Jones JE (1979) How district hospitals see acute colitis. *Br. Med. J.* **iii**, 1226–9.

Chapman RW, Selby WS and Jewell DP (1986) Role of metronidazole in the management of severe ulcerative colitis. *Gut* **27**, 1210–12.

Dickinson RJ, Ashton MG, Axton ATR et al (1980) Controlled trial of intravenous hyperalimentation and total bowel rest as an adjunct to the routine therapy of acute colitis. *Gastroenterology* **79**, 1199–204.

Dickinson RJ, O'Connor HJ, Pinder I et al (1985) Double-blind trial of oral vancomycin as adjunctive treatment in acute exacerbations of ulcerative colitis. *Gut* **26**, 1380–4.

Jewell DP and Baker K (1986) Crohn's disease: corticosteroids and immunosuppressants. In Jewell DP and Ireland A (eds) *Topics in Gastroenterology 14*, chap. 15 Oxford: Blackwell Scientific.

Jewell DP and Truelove SC (1974) Azathioprine in ulcerative colitis: final report on a controlled therapeutic trial. *Br. Med. J.* **2**, 627–30.

Kirk AP and Lennard-Jones JE (1982) Controlled trial of azathioprine in chronic ulcerative colitis. *Br. Med. J.* **284**, 1291–2.

Lennard-Jones JE, Ritchie JK, Hilder W and Spicer CC (1975) Assessment of severity in colitis: a preliminary study. *Gut* **16**, 579–84.

McIntyre PB, Powell-Tuck J, Wood SR et al (1986) Controlled trial of bowel rest in the treatment of severe ulcerative colitis. *Gut* **27**, 481–5.

Meyers S, Sachar DB, Goldberg JD and Janowitz HD (1983) Corticotrophin versus hydrocortisone in the intravenous treatment of ulcerative colitis. *Gastroenterology* **85**, 351–7.

Ritchie JK (1974) Results of surgery for inflammatory bowel disease: a further survey of one hospital region. *Br. Med. J.* **i**, 264–8.

Torsoli A (1981) Toxic megacolon. Part II. Prevention. In Torsoli A (ed.) *Clinics in Gastroenterology*, pp 117–121. London: Saunders.

Truelove SC and Witts LJ (1955) Cortisone in ulcerative colitis—final report on a therapeutic trial. *Br. Med. J.* **2**, 1041–8.

Truelove SC and Witts LJ (1959) Cortisone and corticotrophin in ulcerative colitis. *Br. Med. J.* **i**, 387–94.

Truelove SC and Jewell DP (1974) Intensive intravenous regimen for severe attacks of ulcerative colitis. *Lancet* **i**, 1067–70.

Truelove SC, Watkinson G and Draper G (1962) Comparison of corticosteroids and sulphasalazine therapy in ulcerative colitis. *Br. Med. J.* **2**, 1708–11.

Truelove SC, Willoughby CP, Lee EG and Kettlewell MGW (1978) Further experience in the treatment of severe attacks of ulcerative colitis. *Lancet* **ii**, 1086–8.

Key Developments in Gastroenterology
Edited by P. R. Salmon
© 1988 John Wiley & Sons Ltd

6

Human Immunodeficiency Virus Infection and the Gastroenterologist

Ian V. D. Weller

University College and Middlesex Hospital Medical School, London

Introduction: Acute and Chronic HIV Infection

The acquired immune deficiency syndrome is the end-stage disease of an infection caused by human immunodeficiency virus (HIV, formerly LAV/HTLV-III) (Table 1). The Centers for Disease Control (CDC) definition of AIDS only identifies those infected individuals with certain opportunistic infections, tumours or associated diseases who have developed a progressive irreversible immune deficiency (Centers for Disease Control, 1985). For every case of AIDS, it has been estimated that there are 30 to 300 individuals infected by the virus, who may exhibit acute or chronic features of the infection, or remain asymptomatic (Sivak and Wormser, 1985). The well recognised risk groups reflect the sexual parenteral and perinatal routes of transmission of the virus (Curran et al, 1985).

HIV is a double-stranded RNA retrovirus, which on penetration of a susceptible cell bearing a CD4 antigen receptor (CD = cluster differentiation), makes a DNA copy of itself using a viral reverse transcriptase enzyme. This pro-viral DNA is then incorporated into the host genetic material where it may remain latent or periodically produce new RNA copies. New viral particles are assembled from the RNA, core and envelope proteins. Isolates of HIV show considerable genetic heterogeneity in the envelope gene region (Wong-Staal and Gallo, 1985). A similar virus (LAV-2 or HIV-2) has been isolated from patients with AIDS from West Africa, and from two caucasian homosexual men in Paris. Its morphological and biological features are similar to HIV-1 but it differs in some of its antigenic components, notably the envelope glycoprotein (Clavel et al, 1986). The primary defect induced by HIV infection is in cellular immunity. The CD4 antigen expressed by the helper/inducer subset of T-lymphocytes makes them most susceptible to infection. These lymphocytes have a pivotal role in the immune response. Their depletion and/or a functional abnormality which results from HIV infection leads not only to a loss of cytotoxic T-cell responses but also to a reduction of natural killer cell and monocyte function and B-cell abnormalism with polyclonal B-cell activation, hypergammaglobulinaemia and impairment of specific antibody responses to new antigens (Lawrence, 1985). In addition, HIV has been shown to infect macrophages, B-lymphocyte cell lines and neuroglial cells.

Although most acute infections are asymptomatic, a number of syndromes have been described. The commonest is a non-specific viral or glandular-fever type illness occurring 1–6 weeks after infection. This may present with fever, sweats, malaise, myalgia, arthralgia, sore throat, nausea, headache, diarrhoea, photophobia, a rash and lymphadenopathy (Cooper et al, 1985). An acute meningo-encephalitis and myelopathy have also been described (Carne et al, 1985; Denning et al, 1987).

Seroconversion for anti-HIV occurs typically 4–12 weeks after acute infection, although longer delays in the development of antibody and a persistent antigenaemia in the absence of detectable antibody occur. The antibodies produced to HIV core and envelope proteins in vivo are a readily detectable marker of exposure, but have only weak in vitro neutralising activity and therefore co-exist with latent infection and productive viral replication (Weiss et al, 1985).

The commonest finding in chronic HIV infection is generalised lymphadenopathy. About a third of anti-HIV positive patients fulfil the CDC definition of persistent generalised lymphadenopathy (PGL) with nodes of at least 1 cm in diameter in two extrainguinal sites for three months or more (Jaffe et al, 1985). Many others have lesser degrees of lymphadenopathy. In both categories, the nodes are symmetrical, mobile and non-tender.

Lymph node biopsy is unrewarding in asymptomatic patients revealing only non-specific follicular hyperplasia. If there are constitutional symptoms, such as weight loss or fever, or the nodes are markedly asymmetrical, painful or rapidly enlarging or if there is an extranodal mass or co-existing hilar nodes, then biopsy is essential (Rashleigh-Belcher et al, 1986). This will exclude tumours such as lymphoma or lymphadenopathic Kaposi's sarcoma or an opportunistic infection such as mycobacteria. Tiredness, lethargy, fever and weight loss may occur, without any other identifiable cause. Routine investigation may reveal lymphopenia or an immune neutropenia or thrombocytopenia, but these are not usually severe. The lymphopenia is largely due to the reduction in CD4 positive helper cells.

Minor opportunistic infection is common. Skin conditions encountered include a range of infections: dermatophytic fungal, viral (recalcitrant warts, herpes simplex and herpes zoster) and bacterial (folliculitis, impetigo and furunculosis). The spectrum of other skin disorders ranges from mere dryness to severe seborrhoeic dermatitis.

Table 1 CDC Classification system for HIV infections

Group I	*Acute infection*—will be reclassified following resolution
Group II	*Asymptomatic infection*—must have had no previous signs or symptoms that would have led to classification in groups III or IV
Group III	*Persistent generalised lymphadenopathy*
Group IV	*Other disease* (subgroup classification independent of lymphadenopahy)
Subgroups A	*Constitutional disease* (fever > one month, weight loss > 10% base line, diarrhoea > one month)
B	*Neurological disease* (dementia, myelopathy, peripheral neuropathy)
C	*Secondary infectious diseases* C1 those specified in CDC surveillance definition C2 others: oral hairy leucoplakia, multidermatomal, herpes zoster, recurrent salmonella bacteraemia, nocardiosis, tuberculosis, oral candida
D	*Secondary cancers*—Kaposi's sarcoma, non-Hodgkin's lymphoma, primary cerebral lymphoma
E	*Other conditions*

N.B. 1. Patients in groups II and III may be subclassified on the basis of laboratory abnormalities, e.g. lymphopenia, ↓ T helper lymphocytes, etc.

2. Patients in group IV A + B must have no concurrent illness or condition to explain findings other than HIV infection.

3. Group IV E is defined as the presence of other clinical findings or diseases not classifiable by the above scheme which might be attributed to HIV infection, e.g. chronic lymphoid interstitial pneumonitis, patients with constitutional symptoms, infectious diseases or tumours not meeting the criteria for groups IV A, C and D.

The risk of progression to AIDS from published studies ranges from 7 to 30% over 3–4 years (Carne et al, 1987a). However, prospective cohort studies only represent a short period of observation from which to draw conclusions about the natural history of HIV infection. Prognostic markers for disease progression have been identified from these studies (Loveday and Weller, 1987). Clinical features include constitutional symptoms, oral candida, leukoplakia and herpes zoster. Haematological and immunological abnormalities include cytopenias, particularly progressive depletion of CD4 positive lymphocytes, anaemia, a raised β_2 microglobulin, a raised ESR, impairment of in vitro gamma interferon production, lymphocyte responses to pokeweed mitogen and perhaps specific cellular responses to HIV. More recently a decline in titre or disappearance of serum anti-P24 (the antibody to HIV core protein) and the appearance of P24 have been shown to antedate the development of the full-blown syndrome (Weber et al, 1987a). The CDC have recently proposed a classification scheme for HIV infection related to our present understanding of disease progression (Centers for Disease Control, 1986) (Table 1). Amongst a sub-population of homosexual men, the risk of HIV infection has brought about a change in sexual

Table 2   Sexually transmitted infections of the gastrointestinal tract and liver

Symptoms	Sigmoidoscopy		Organisms
Anorectal	Proctitis and/or ulceration		*Neisseria gonorrhoea* Herpes simplex virus (HSV) *Chlamydia trachomatis* *Treponema pallidum*
Anorectal and enteric	Proctocolitis		*Campylobacter* spp *Shigella* spp *Chlamydia trachomatis* (LGV) *Entamoeba histolytica*
Enteric	Normal		*Giardia lamblia*
Hepatitis	—	*Common:*	Hepatitis A virus (HAV) Hepatitis B virus (HBV)
		Rare:	Hepatitis C virus (NANB) Hepatitis D virus (δ) Epstein–Barr virus (EBV) Cytomegalovirus (CMV)

behaviour with a reduction in the number of partners and 'safer' sexual practices. This has resulted in a reduction of common sexually transmitted diseases, many of which affect the gastrointestinal tract and liver (Table 2) (Carne et al, 1987b; Weller, 1985, 1986). However, a variety of new syndromes with a varied aetiology affecting both systems are being recognised as complications of HIV infection, many of which fulfil the criteria for AIDS (Table 3).

Clinical Syndromes

Retrosternal discomfort – dysphagia

Oral and oesophageal candidiasis was one of the features documented in the first cases of AIDS. It can be asymptomatic or cause oropharangeal discomfort with oesophageal involvement, retrosternal chest pain and discomfort and/or difficulty on swallowing. Oral candidiasis alone does not fulfil the criteria for AIDS. Oesophageal involvement is best demonstrated preferably by culture or biopsy at endoscopy, although plaques of candida can often be demonstrated on barium swallow (Figure 1). Ulceration may be focal or diffuse. Both cytomegalovirus and herpes simplex virus may also cause a similar pattern of ulceration in the oesophagus, but also in the stomach and duodenum, and it may be difficult to differentiate them with barium studies (Table 3). However, since oesophageal candidiasis is so common (Figure 1) a pragmatic approach in a patient with oral candida and oesophageal symptoms would be to treat empirically for candidiasis and to only proceed to endoscopy should there be no response. One major drawback of this approach is that biopsy or culture proven oesophageal candidiasis is required for the diagnosis of AIDS.

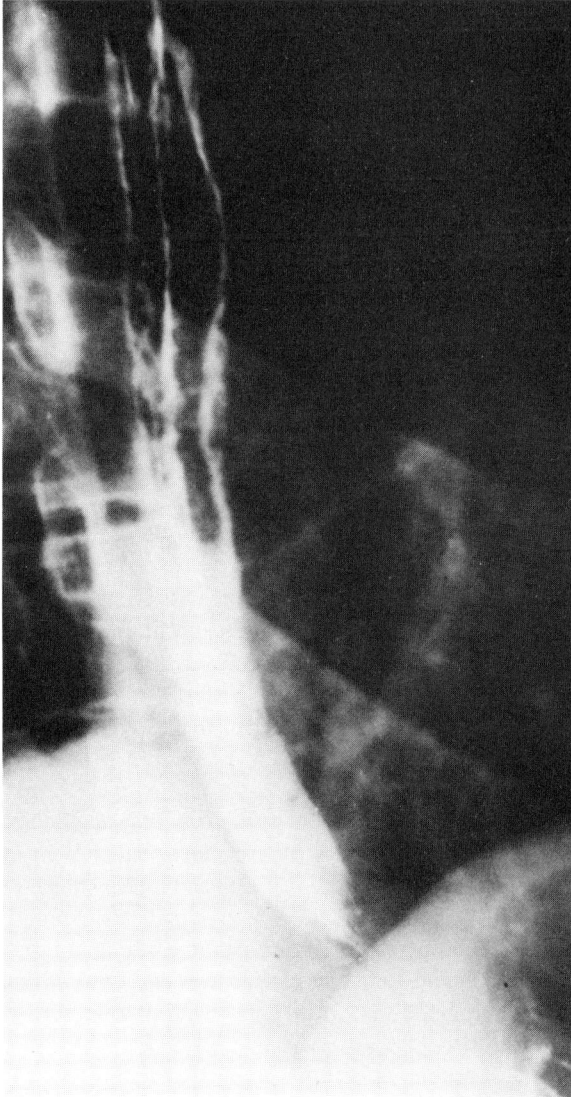

Figure 1. Oesophageal candidiasis.

Table 3   Conditions affecting the gastrointestinal tract and liver in AIDS

Syndrome	Causes
Retrosternal discomfort/dysphagia	Candidiasis Cytomegalovirus (CMV) Herpes simplex virus (HSV)
Diarrhoea/weight loss/malabsorption	Unknown—enteropathy Cryptosporidium (*Isospora belli* and microsporidia) CMV/HSV Mycobacteria Enteric bacteria—salmonella, campylobacter Neoplasia
Hepatitis/cholestasis	Mycobacteria Cryptosporidium Cytomegalovirus Cryptococcus neoformans Drug induced
Neoplasia and miscellaneous	Kaposi's sarcoma Lymphoma Hairy leukoplakia Recalcitrant anorectal warts Squamous oral/anal carcinoma

Diarrhoea, malabsorption and weight loss

Diarrhoea is a common symptom of patients with chronic HIV infection with and without other manifestations of AIDS. In many cases a cause is not found. Symptomatic treatment is all there is to offer. An enteropathy with villous atrophy and malabsorption has been described, but the prevalence of this condition and its aetiology have yet to be determined (Kotler et al, 1984).

Cryptosporidium is a coccidian protozoal parasite and probably the commonest pathogen isolated in AIDS patients with diarrhoea and certainly the commonest of the protozoal causes of diarrhoea, which also include *Isospora belli* and microsporidia (DeHovitz et al, 1986; Dobbins and Weinstein, 1985; Modigliani et al, 1985). Cryptosporidium is widely distributed in the animal kingdom. In immunocompetent human hosts it produces a transient diarrhoeal illness. In HIV-infected hosts it can cause transient, intermittent or persistent diarrhoea, ranging from loose stool to watery diarrhoea, with colic and severe fluid and electrolyte loss.

The first reports of human infection were in 1976 in a three-year-old child with a severe self-limiting illness and a 39-year-old man with bullous phemphigoid and ulcerative colitis on immunosuppressive therapy. The diarrhoea resolved with immunosuppressant withdrawal. Subsequently cases were described in other immunocompromised patients (Nime et al, 1976; Sloper et al, 1982). By 1982, 21 patients with AIDS and a severe protracted diarrhoea caused by cryptosporidium had been reported to the CDC and by March 1984 a further 91 patients had been documented (Centers for Disease Control, 1984). In reports before 1978, oocysts of cryptosporidium were not identified in the stool and diagnosis rested on demonstrating the intermediate forms on biopsy material. However, in recent years improved staining techniques on stool specimens have allowed an easier diagnosis and have enhanced our understanding of the disease.

In severe cases it presents as a protracted watery, non-bloody diarrhoea often lasting many months before diagnosis with weight loss and malabsorption. In severe cases patients may pass up to 10 litres a day.

Following ingestion of the oocyst the asexual and sexual life cycles occur in the bowel. The various forms of cryptosporidium, such as the trophozoites, schizonts and macrogametocytes, have been found in biopsy material from the pharynx to the rectum of infected humans but infection seems to be most severe in the small bowel. The organism does not appear to be invasive. There may be varying degrees of villous atrophy (Soave et al, 1984). Contrast studies are often normal, but may show a non-specific malabsorption pattern in the small bowel.

Previously, diagnosis rested on obtaining biopsy material, but with the small size of the intermediate forms they can easily be missed. Oocysts (4–5 μm) can be found in the stool. In AIDS patients, direct smears of unconcentrated faecal samples may be all that is required with iodine or modified acid-fast stains. If these fail to reveal the oocysts then concentration is required, such as a modified Sheathers flotation method followed by bright-field microscopy or staining (Ma and Soave, 1983).

Herpes virus infections

Two members of the herpes virus group have been associated with gastro-intestinal disease in AIDS patients: herpes simplex virus (HSV) and cytomegalovirus (CMV). These viruses have a number of common properties. Following primary infection the viruses remain latent in their host—a state where the functional viral genome persists but there is no active replication. Reactivation with a high level of viral replication may occur at any time following primary infection and this may or may not be accompanied by clinical manifestations (Figure 2). Primary infection and reactivation of infection may cause severe disease in the immunocompromised. Serious disseminated infections occur in organ transplant recipients with involvement of many organs, especially if primary infection occurs. The diagnosis largely rests with culture of the virus from the lesions. However, herpes viruses may be shed from a large number of epithelial surfaces in immunocompromised hosts and the presence of the virus may not necessarily indicate an aetiological link with the epithelial lesion.

In AIDS, herpes viruses CMV and HSV can cause focal or diffuse ulceration of the gut, from the mouth to the anus. Most commonly, HSV causes mucocutaneous lesions at the upper and the lower ends of the gastrointestinal tract, whilst CMV may mimic inflammatory bowel disease.

Primary infection with HSV is a common cause of non-gonococcal proctitis in homosexual men. HSV was isolated in as many as 23% of homosexual men presenting with anorectal pain, rectal discharge, which is sometimes bloody, and tenesmus (Goodell et al, 1983). Neurological symptoms such as difficulty with micturition, constipation, paraesthesiae and pain in the distribution of the sacral roots may occur. Common clinical findings are perianal ulceration, inguinal lymphadenopathy and ulcers in the distal rectum. This can be severe but is a self-

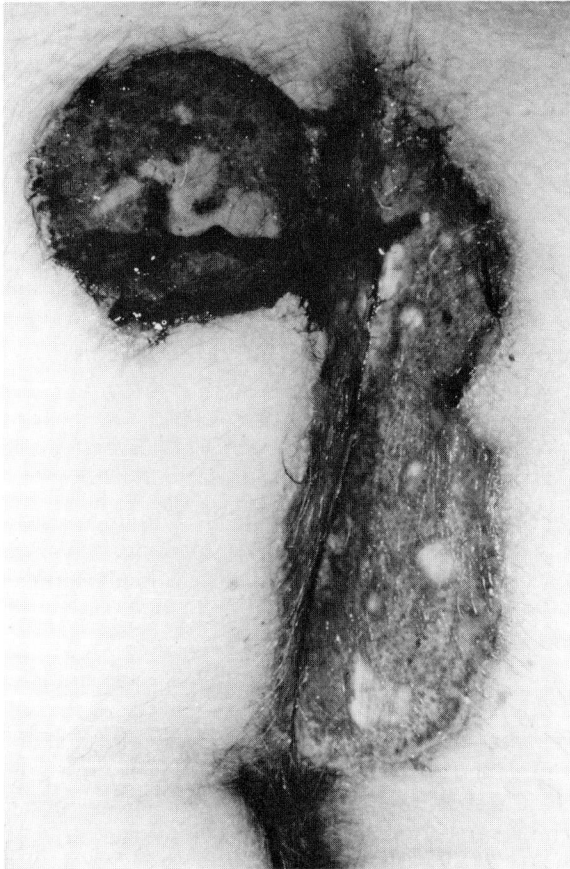

Figure 2. Severe mucocutaneous ulceration caused by herpes simplex virus.

limiting illness. The lesions or recurrences are often asymptomatic or mild but prospective studies following primary infection are still required.

With progressive chronic HIV infection recurrences may become increasingly frequent and/or severe. In AIDS large, deep ulcers of the perianal area occur (Figure 2). Similar but smaller lesions may occur around the mouth. Perianal ulceration often occurs in the setting of a chronically ill patient, often with other opportunistic infections and severe weight loss, and must be differentiated from pressure sores. The ulcers tend not to occur on pressure points and HSV is readily isolated from them. Ulceration may also occur in the oesophagus and bronchial tree (Macher, 1984).

Several studies have demonstrated a high prevalence of antibodies to CMV (94%) and isolation of the virus from urine or semen in 7–15% of asymptomatic homosexual men. However, most primary infections would seem to be asymptomatic, although occasionally a Paul-Bunnel negative infectious mononucleosis syndrome can occur. Gut involvement by CMV has been described in other immunosuppressed patients limited to isolated ulcerated segments, usually large bowel, with perforation or occasionally massive haemorrhage described. In AIDS, CMV has been associated with a syndrome which can mimic acute inflammatory bowel disease, with abdominal pain, fever and diarrhoea (Weber et al, 1987b). There may be diffuse or segmental ulceration (Balthazar et al, 1985). Toxic dilatation, perforation and haemorrhage have been described. Diagnosis is made by endoscopy with biopsy and culture. Histologically there is a non-specific inflammation, with dense, round (Owl's eye) intranuclear inclusion bodies in swollen cells. These inclusions are seen most readily in the vascular endothelium of inflamed areas suggesting that the colitis is caused by a virally induced vasculitis (Frager et al, 1986). Barium studies may reveal ulceration but may not differentiate CMV infection from other causes of ulceration such as HSV, Kaposi's sarcoma or lymphoma (see below). Disseminated CMV infection often occurs as a terminal event in AIDS patients and there is no specific therapy of proven value.

Atypical mycobacteria of the avium intracellulare complex are ubiquitous organisms with little virulence for the immunocompetent host. Disseminated infection occurs in AIDS with multi-organ involvement. Gastrointestinal infection may be associated with fever, weight loss, diarrhoea and malabsorption. Diagnosis can be made by acid-fast staining of the stool and/or biopsy material or blood and tissue culture. Gut involvement may mimic Whipple's disease in appearance (Rotterdam and Sommers, 1985). The small bowel shows prominent folds, with PAS positive foamy macrophages, containing the organisms, and filling the lamina propria. The bacteria are acid fast, unlike those of Whipple's disease. M tuberculosis infection of the bowel does occur, but is less common. Campylobacter and salmonella species infections may cause diarrhoea but the latter more commonly present as a pyrexia of unknown origin (PUO) with bacteraemia (Nadelman et al, 1985; Jarrett and

Zeegen, 1986). As with other infections in patients with AIDS, relapses are common following cessation of appropriate antibiotic therapy.

Hepatitis and cholestasis

Hepatitis in AIDS patients may present with fever, abdominal pain, hepatomegaly and abnormal liver function tests, in particular a raised alkaline phosphatase. In the absence of dilated bile ducts on ultrasound needle biopsy most commonly demonstrates a granulomatous hepatitis, usually caused by atypical mycobacteria rather than M tuberculosis. Atypical mycobacteria may be demonstrated on acid-fast staining or culture in the absence of granulomata. *Cryptococcus neoformans* may also be involved (Orenstein et al, 1985; Gordon et al, 1986). The herpes viruses may also occasionally cause hepatitis as part of a disseminated infection. With the multiple therapies being employed, a drug induced hepatitis must always be considered in an AIDS patient with abnormal liver function tests.

More recently acalculous cholecystitis and cholangitis have been described with an endoscopic retrograde cholangiographic picture similar to primary sclerosing cholangitis with strictures and dilatation of the biliary tree (Figure 3). Dilatation and irregularities of the pancreatic duct have also been reported. Histologically there is non-specific inflammation and ulceration. Cryptosporidium and CMV have been demonstrated and/or isolated and implicated as a cause of this syndrome. Gram-negative bacteria and candida have also been cultured (Margulis et al, 1986; Kavin et al, 1986; Cockerill et al, 1986; Gross et al, 1986).

Vaccination programmes using plasma derived hepatitis B vaccine are in progress in the developing and developed world in risk groups with high HIV attack rates. A recent study has shown a suboptimal response in asymptomatic anti-HIV positive homosexual men with only 50% developing detectable anti-HBS (Carne et al, 1987c). HIV may have a considerable impact on the efficacy of this and other vaccines and the public health, especially in the Third World.

Tumours

Kaposi's sarcoma (KS)

Prior to the epidemic of HIV, KS was a rare tumour in North America and Europe with an annual incidence of 0.02 to 0.06 per 100 000. It occurred mainly in men over 50 years of age, of Jewish or Mediterranean ancestry. This classical form of the disease is usually confined to the lower limbs, runs an indolent course and responds well to radiotherapy or chemotherapy (Volberding et al, 1983; Safai and Weiss, 1984). The tumour occurs in immunocompromised

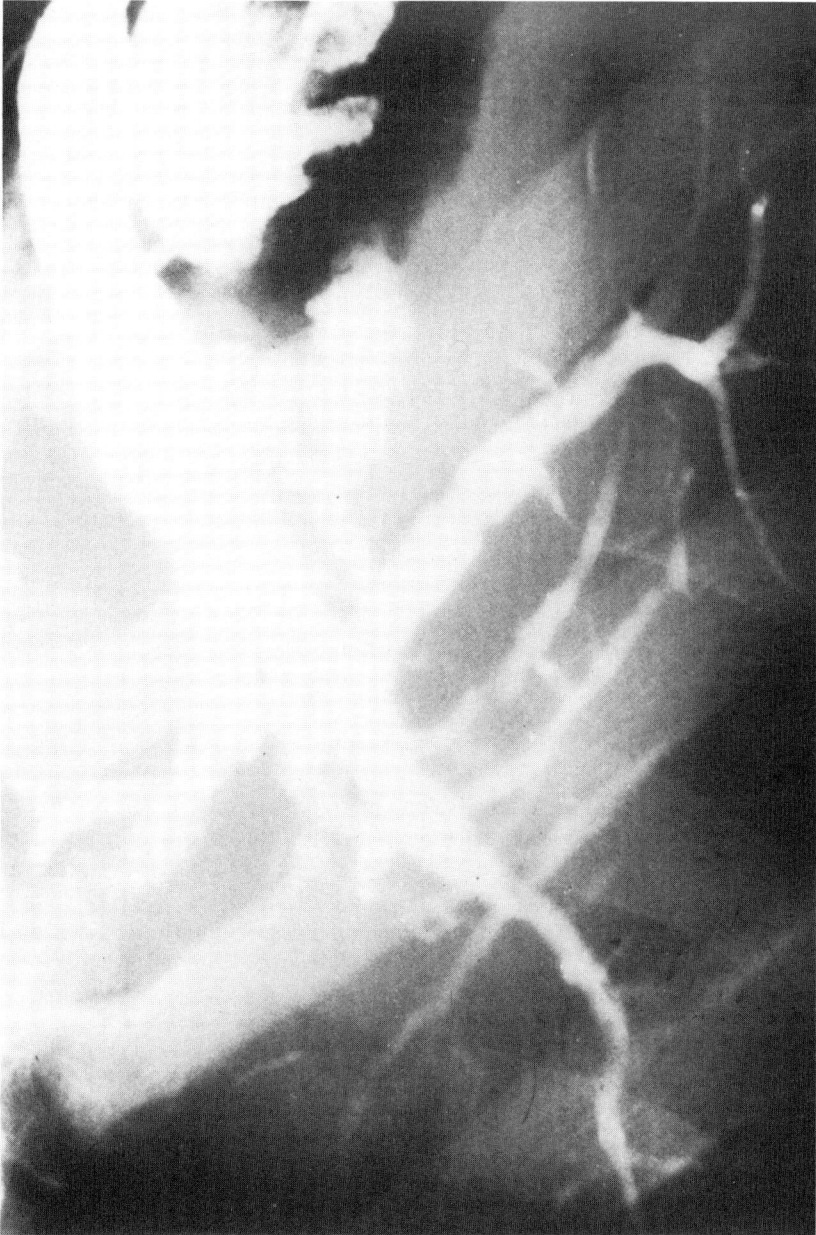

Figure 3. Cholangitis: dilated common bile duct with stricture at lower end and irregularities of extra- and intrahepatic ducts.

patients, especially renal allograft recipients in whom it is more aggressive. Withdrawal of immunosuppression in this situation leads to tumour regression in as many as 50% (Harwood et al, 1979).

However, in Central Africa, KS is a common tumour and accounts for some 9% of malignancies. The majority resemble the classical form seen in North America and Europe but a more aggressive disease with lymph node and visceral involvement has been described in children and young adults.

KS alone in the developed world is the second commonest presenting feature of AIDS (26% of reported cases) after pneumocystis carinii pneumonia (51% of cases), 8% having both. The tumour is significantly more common amongst homosexual men compared with the other groups at risk, who present more frequently with opportunistic infections. Its aetiology is unknown but this observation might suggest that a sexually transmitted agent other than HIV may be involved. Cytomegalovirus infection has been implicated in both the classical and HIV related disease on the basis of seroepidemiological studies and the finding of virus particles and nucleic acid in tumour tissue. The role for CMV is unclear. Other workers have not confirmed these findings and if present the virus may only be a passenger. A genetic predisposition with a higher frequency of HLA-DR5 in both classical and HIV related disease has also been described.

HIV related KS is characterised by widespread skin, mucous membrane, visceral and lymph node involvement (Friedman-Kien et al, 1982). Skin lesions are the most common presenting complaint. They appear as pink or red macules or violaceous plaques and nodules on the face, trunk or limbs. Early skin lesions may be difficult to differentiate from other benign skin conditions such as granulomas, bruises, naevi, dermatofibromata, secondary syphilis or lichen planus. Histologically, the tumours consist of spindle-shaped cells arranged in broad bands with vascular slits between and extravasation of erythrocytes between the spindle cells. The histological appearances of HIV related and classical KS are indistinguishable.

The gastrointestinal tract is one of the commonest internal organs to be involved. If upper and lower gastrointestinal endoscopy is performed at presentation, lesions will be demonstrated in about 40% of patients. At post mortem they are present in more than 70%. Involvement of the hard palate and alveolar ridges, oropharynx, oesophagus, stomach, duodenum, colon and rectum have been demonstrated (Figure 4). Lesions resemble the range seen in the skin from small, flat telangiectatic lesions, not well demonstrated by contrast studies and only seen at endoscopy to larger nodular or polypoid lesions. Endoscopic biopsy has a high false negative rate with only 23% of suspicious lesions being confirmed histologically because of their predominant position deep to the submucosa (Friedman et al, 1985).

The median survival from diagnosis is about 30 months with some patients running a more rapid, fulminant course and others remaining well for several years with minimal cutaneous disease. Supervening opportunistic infection is the

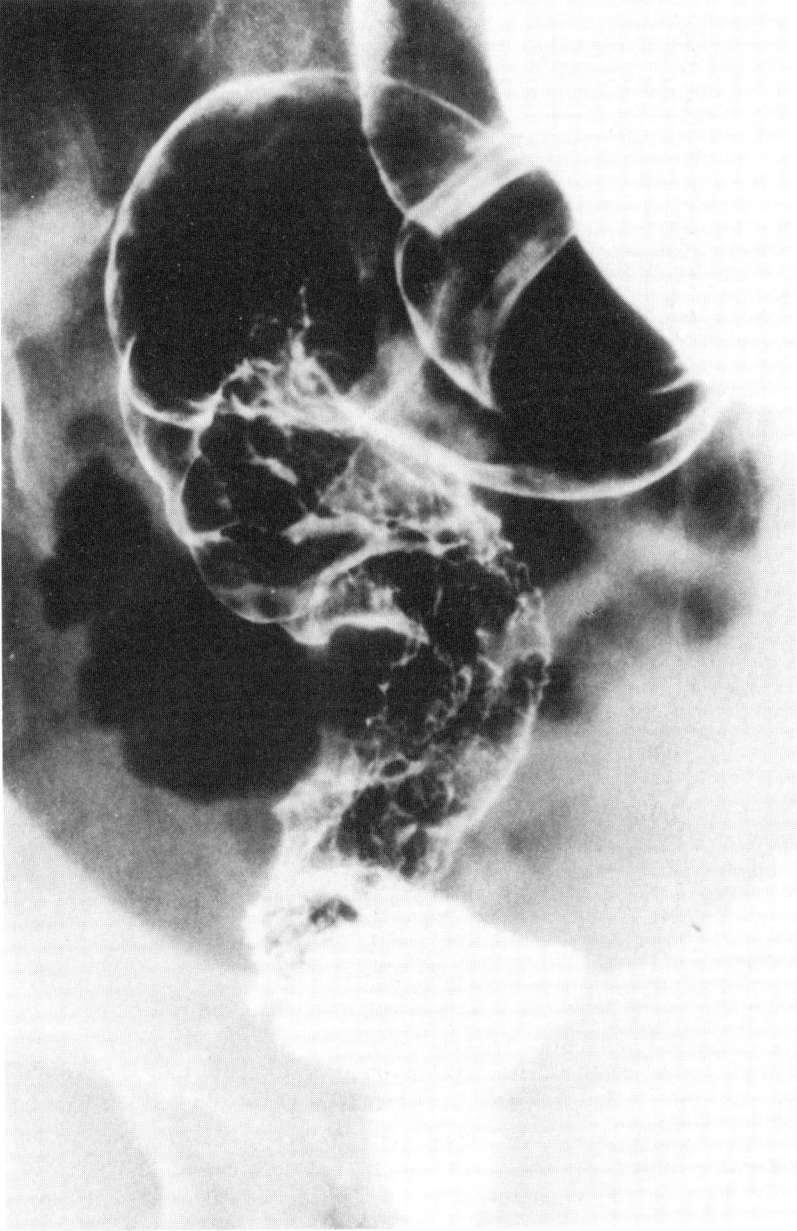

Figure 4. Kaposi's sarcoma of the rectum.

Table 4 Staging of Kaposi's sarcoma

		Classical	HIV-related
Stage I	(A + B)	Local indolent	Limited cutaneous (one anatomical region)
Stage II	(A + B)	Local aggressive	Disseminated cutaneous ($>$ one anatomical region)
Stage III	(A + B)	Generalised mucocutaneous/ lymphadenopathic	Visceral only (e.g. lymph node/GI tract)
Stage IV	(A + B)	Visceral	Cutaneous and visceral

A = No symptoms
B = Non-specific symptoms, e.g. fever and weight loss.

commonest problem in patients with KS alone, and the usual terminal event. Complications from involvement of the gut are unusual. Haemorrhage from lesions either acute or chronic leading to iron deficiency anaemia may occur. Several cases of KS presenting as an acute inflammatory bowel like syndrome with diarrhoea and ulceration on barium enema have also been described (Weber et al, 1985). A protein-losing enteropathy may also occur.

Except for these circumstances, endoscopy is not routinely required to demonstrate visceral involvement if the diagnosis is made on the basis of mucocutaneous lesions. However, it is used in clinical trials to adequately stage the extent of the tumour. The staging system used for classical KS is inappropriate because the locally indolent and aggressive forms of tumour are rare and an alternative staging system has been suggested (Table 4).

Lymphoma

Early studies identified small numbers of homosexual men with non-Hodgkin's lymphoma developing in a setting of PGL, opportunistic infections and KS. According to the original definition of AIDS, homosexual men with lymphomas other than primary cerebral could not be notified as AIDS because lymphomas were considered to be a known cause of immunosuppression. However, Cancer Registry data in San Francisco and Los Angeles indicated up to a threefold rise in high-grade lymphomas in young never-married men in 1983 and the characteristics of 90 such cases in homosexual men were reported (Ziegler et al, 1984). The tumours are of B-cell origin and may present de novo, in a setting of prodromal lymphadenophy, opportunistic infection or Kaposi's sarcoma. The majority of patients in this series presented with extranodal involvement, predominantly in the central nervous system, bone marrow and gut (Table 5).

Table 5 Extranodal sites of non-Hodgkin's lymphoma in 88 patients

CNS	Brain mass:	21
	Other:	24
Bone marrow		30
GI tract		22
Lung		8
Liver		8
Skin		7
Other		7

Modified from Ziegler et al (1984)

The survival and response to treatment was poor. These features are similar to those of the generalised and aggressive KS of AIDS. Non-Hodgkin's lymphoma is now recognised as another manifestation of AIDS but the mechanisms involved in the transition from the follicular hyperplasia of PGL with polyclonal B-cell activation through to B-cell lymphoma and the role of HIV and other human T-cell tropic viruses and Esptein–Barr virus (EBV) have yet to be fully determined.

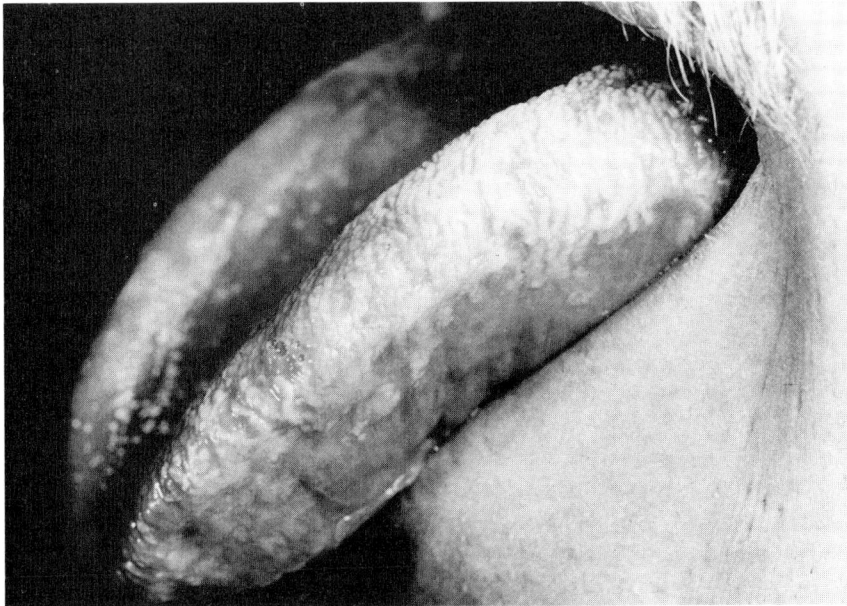

Figure 5. Leukoplakia of the tongue.

Other conditions

The recently described hairy leukoplakia presents as greyish-white lesions, typically on the lateral borders of the tongue, and does not respond to antifungal therapy (Figure 5). Histologically there are keratin projections resembling hairs, koilocytosis and mild atypia. Its cause is unknown but BV DNA has been demonstrated in these lesions by hybridisation with specific probes and there have been anecdotal reports of response to acyclovir (Greenspan et al, 1985; Friedman-Kien, 1986).

Recalcitrant anogenital warts are a common problem in homosexual men with chronic HIV infection and recurrence rates with all forms of therapy are high. There have been anecdotal reports of squamous oral and anal carcinoma in anti-HIV positive homosexual men and the role of human papillomavirus (HPV) and perhaps other viruses have yet to be elucidated (Conant et al, 1982).

Treatment

The therapy of HIV infection has been largely limited to the treatment of its malignant and infectious complications. Cytotoxic therapy for the tumours may lead to further immunosuppression and the risk of life-threatening opportunistic infection. Most of the infections are due to reactivation of latent organisms in the host or in some cases to ubiquitous organisms to which we are continuously exposed. The treatment of these infections tends to suppress rather than eradicate organisms, so relapse is common when therapy is stopped. Furthermore, the side effects of many of the drugs used do not easily facilitate the long-term therapy that is required.

Kaposi's sarcoma

The median survival from time of diagnosis, for patients with KS alone, is substantially better than those with opportunistic infection (33 vs 8 months). In the absence of any evidence for improved survival with early therapy, the first lesions of KS may require no treatment. Local radiotherapy can be used for treatment of mucocutaneous lesions for cosmetic reasons and for larger lesions causing local complications, such as those in the oropharynx. Systemic chemotherapy is used in generalised mucocutaneous disease with or without visceral involvement. Various single agent and combined cytotoxic regimens have been used with their many side effects, risk of further immunosuppression and reactivation of latent infection. Lymphoblastoid and recombinant human alpha interferons have been used with a few complete remissions; 30 to 40% of patients have partial remissions with this treatment, but severe side effects are common with constitutional symptoms and cytopenias. At present the best that we should expect with any form of systemic therapy is a temporary, partial remission at considerable cost to the patient in terms of adverse effects and with no evidence yet that the treatment will alter the long-term prognosis. Many centres therefore have a conservative policy for the use of such therapy in most cases of Kaposi's sarcoma.

Viral infections

Herpes simplex infections respond to oral acyclovir (Mindel et al, 1984). Prophylactic treatment (200 mg q.d.s.) may be required as severe, frequent recurrences are common in chronic HIV infection short of AIDS. Intravenous acyclovir is preferred for the severe persistent mucocutaneous infections.

Ganciclovir (DHPG), like acyclovir, is an acyclic analogue of deoxyguanosine. It has shown promising results in uncontrolled studies in the treatment of cytomegalovirus infection (Collaborative DHPG Treatment Study Group, 1986). Maintenance therapy is required and even then relapse or progression may occur. Phosphonoformate (Foscarnet) has also been used in CMV infections with some success (Weber et al, 1987b). It is a pyrophosphate analogue and inhibits polymerase enzymes, but it has to be given as a continuous intravenous infusion. Intravenous therapy with both agents is a major drawback to antiviral maintenance therapy but many patients are being maintained without complications at home, using Hickman catheters.

Protozoal infections

Cryptosporidiosis may respond to spiramycin (1 g q.d.s.) (Portnoy et al, 1984) or a combination of quinine and clindamycin, but reported success is anecdotal. Symptoms and excretion of cysts may be intermittent and so spontaneous remission may occur. There are also anecdotal reports of a response to interleukin 2 (Kern and Dietrich, 1985). Symptomatic treatment with codeine phosphate, loperamide and other drugs may be the only effective measure. Isosporiasis responds well to co-trimoxazole (two tablets q.d.s.) for 10 days, but relapses occur in 50% of cases with cessation of treatment (De Hovitz et al, 1986).

Bacterial infections

Salmonella species infections respond to treatment with appropriate antibiotics, but relapses of enteritis and/or bacteraemia are common.

Diarrhoea may respond to metronidazole, even in the absence of recognised pathogens in the stool. Symptomatic treatment with codeine phosphate, loperamide and other drugs can be used, and may be the only effective treatment for cryptosporidiosis. Mycobacterium tuberculosis is treated conventionally. The atypical organisms are resistant to conventional antituberculous therapy. Ansamycin (a rifamycin derivative) and clofazimine (an anti-leprosy compound) are among the agents being tried, having been shown to have some in vitro activity, but the treatment of patients with disseminated infection has been largely unsuccessful. Until a specific therapy is found the exact pathogenic role of these organisms in the many clinical syndromes of AIDS will be difficult to elucidate.

Fungal infections

Oral candida is often asymptomatic in its early stages and may not require therapy. In more severe infections, local treatment with frequent nystatin suspension or pastilles or amphotericin lozenges can be used. Systemic therapy with ketoconazole 200–400 mg orally daily may be required, and is the drug of choice for oesophageal candidiasis. Long-term therapy may be required to prevent recurrences and liver function tests should be monitored. Cryptococcal and other systemic fungal infections require treatment with amphotericin with or without flucytosine for a minimum of six weeks.

Antivirals

The ideal antiviral agent should be specific, orally absorbed and cross the blood/brain barrier. It should also be free from adverse effects, since the best we can anticipate is suppression of productive viral replication with the problem of latently infected cells remaining. Theoretically, inhibition of productive viral replication may allow some recovery of immune function perhaps encouraging regression of tumours and elimination of the conditions favouring opportunistic infections.

A variety of potential targets for antiviral therapy have now been identified from a better understanding of the replicative cycle and molecular biology of HIV. Most efforts are being focused on specific inhibitors of the HIV reverse transcriptase enzyme.

The most promising group of reverse transcriptase inhibitors are the 2′, 3′ dideoxynucleoside analogues. 3′-azido-3′-deoxythymidine (Zidovudine, formerly azidothymidine, AZT) has been shown to have considerable in vitro activity against HIV. It is a competitive inhibitor of reverse transcriptase and a DNA chain terminator.

Zidovudine is orally absorbed and cerebrospinal fluid levels are approximately 50% of corresponding plasma levels. In a double-blind randomised controlled clinical trial of oral therapy (250 mg orally 4-hourly for six months) in 280 patients with past pneumocystis carinii pneumonia or severe symptomatic chronic HIV infection (AIDS-related complex), it has been shown to significantly reduce mortality and morbidity and decrease episodes of opportunistic infection (Fischl et al, 1987; Richman et al, 1977). There were significant improvements in some immunological parameters and a significant antiviral action was demonstrated by a decrease in serum P24 (viral core protein). Small uncontrolled studies have shown improvement in neurological disease. Side effects include a megaloblastic anaemia, neutropenia, nausea, insomnia and myalgia. Dideoxycytidine is undergoing phase one studies and preliminary data suggest that it is a more potent inhibitor of HIV on a molar basis and is less toxic.

Controlled trials of Zidovudine and other antiviral agents alone or in combination to reduce toxicity and improve efficacy are planned, in asymptomatic patients with laboratory markers which predict more rapid progression to AIDS. Because of the demonstrated efficacy of Zidovudine in patients with AIDS-related complex this will be used as an end point in such trials. If found to be beneficial in this situation and provided that side effects are minimal, controlled trials will then be carried out very early in HIV infection, even at the point of seroconversion.

Future aims will be not only to combine antiviral agents but also antiviral and immunomodulatory therapies (if effective and beneficial examples of the latter are found) in large placebo controlled trials. Enhancement of the immune response to HIV may be one way of eradicating the virus from some of its latent sites.

Acknowledgements

Dr I.V.D. Weller is a Wellcome Trust Senior Lecturer in Infectious Diseases.

References

Balthazar EJ, Megibow AJ, Fazzini E, Opulencia JF and Engel I (1985) Cytomegalovirus colitis in AIDS: radiographic findings in 11 patients. *Radiology* **155**, 585–9.

Carne CA, Tedder RS, Smith A et al (1985) Acute encephalopathy coincident with seroconversion for anti-HTLV III. *Lancet* **ii**, 1206–1208.

Carne CA, Weller IVD, Loveday C and Adler MW (1987a) From persistent generalised lymphadenopathy to AIDS: who will progress? *Br. Med. J.* **294**, 868–9.

Carne CA, Weller IVD, Johnson AM et al (1987b) Prevalence of antibodies to human immunodeficiency virus, gonorrhoea rates and changed sexual behaviour in homosexual men in London. *Lancet* **i**, 656–8.

Carne CA, Weller IVD, Waite J et al (1987) Impaired responsiveness of homosexual men with antibodies to Human Immunodeficiency Virus (HIV) to plasma derived Hepatitis B vaccine. *Br. Med. J.* **294**, 866–8.

Centers for Disease Control (1984) Update: treatment of cryptosporidiosis in patients with acquired immunodeficiency syndrome (AIDS). *MMWR* **33**, 117–9.

Centers for Disease Control (1985) Revision of the case definition of the acquired immunodeficiency syndrome for national reporting—United States. *MMWR* **34**, 373–5.

Centers for Disease Control (1986) Classification system for Human T-lymphotropic virus type III/Lymphadenopathy-associated virus infections. *MMWR* **35**, 334–9.

Clavel F, Guetard D, Brun-Vezinet F et al (1986) Isolation of a new human retrovirus from West African patients with AIDS. *Science* **233**, 343–6.

Cockerill FR, Hurley DV, Malagelada JR et al (1986) Polymicrobial cholangitis and Kaposi's sarcoma in blood product transfusion-related acquired immune deficiency syndrome. *Am. J. Med.* **80**, 1237–41.

Collaborative DHPG Treatment Study Group (1986) Treatment of serious cytomegalovirus infections with 9-(1, 3-Dihydroxy-2-propoxymethyl) guanine in patients with AIDS and other immunodeficiencies. *N. Eng. J. Med.* **314**, 801–5.

Cooper DA, Gold J, Maclean P et al (1985) Acute AIDS retrovirus infection. *Lancet* **i**, 537–40.

Conant MA, Volberding P, Fletcher V, Lozarda FL and Silverman S (1982) Squamous cell carcinoma in sexual partner of Kaposi's sarcoma patient. *Lancet* **i**, 286.

Curran JW, Meade Morgan W, Hardy AM, Jaffe HW, Darrow WW, Dowdle WR (1985) The Epidemiology of AIDS: Current Status and Future Prospects. *Science* **229**, 1352–7.

DeHovitz JA, Pape JW, Boncy M and Johnson WD (1986) Clinical manifestations and therapy of isospora belli infection in patients with the acquired immunodeficiency syndrome. *N. Eng. J. Med.* **315**, 87–90.

Denning DW, Anderson J, Rudge P and Smith H (1987) Acute myelopathy associated with primary infection with human immunodeficiency virus. *Br. Med. J.* **294**, 143–4.

Dobbins WV III and Weinstein WM (1985) Electron microscopy of the intestine and rectum in the acquired immunodeficiency syndrome. *Gastroenterology* **88**, 738–49.

Fischl MA, Rickman DD and Grieco MH (1987) The efficacy of Azidothymidine (AZT) in the treatment of patients with AIDS and AIDS-related complex. *N. Eng. J. Med.* **317**, 185–91.

Frager DH, Frager JD, Wolf EL et al (1986) Cytomegalovirus colitis in acquired immune deficiency syndrome: radiologic spectrum. *Gastrointest. Radiol.* **11**, 241–6.

Friedman-Kien AE (1986) Viral origin of hairy leucoplakia. *Lancet* **ii**, 694.

Friedman-Kien A, Laubenstein LJ, Rubinstein P et al (1982) Disseminated Kaposi's sarcoma in homosexual men. *Ann. Intern. Med.* **96**, 693–700.

Friedman SL, Wright TL and Altman DF (1985) Gastrointestinal Kaposi's sarcoma in patients with acquired immunodeficiency syndrome. Endoscopic and autopsy findings. *Gastroenterology* **89**, 102–8.

Goodell SE, Quinn TC, Mkrtichian E et al (1983) Herpes simplex proctitis in homosexual men: clinical, sigmoidoscopic and histopathological features. *N. Eng. J. Med.* **308**, 868–71.

Gordon SC, Reddy KR, Gould EE et al (1986) The spectrum of liver disease in the acquired immunodeficiency syndrome. *J. Hepatol.* **2(3)**, 475–84.

Greenspan JS, Greenspan D, Lennette ET et al (1985) Replication of Epstein-Barr virus within the epithelial cells of oral 'hairy' leucoplakia, and AIDS-associated lesion. *N. Eng. J. Med.* **313**, 1564–71.

Gross TL, Wheat J, Bartlett M and O'Connor KW (1986) AIDS and multiple system involvement with cryptosporidium. *Am. J. Gastroenterol.* **81(6)**, 456–8.

Harwood AR, Osoba D and Hofstader SL (1979) Kaposi's sarcoma in recipients of renal transplants. *Am. J. Med.* **67**, 759–65.

Jaffe HW, Darrow WW, Edenberg DF et al (1985) The acquired immunodeficiency syndrome in a cohort of homosexual men. A six year follow up study. *Ann. Int. Med.* **103**, 210–4.

Jarrett DRJ and Zeegen R (1986) Recurrent typhoid in an HTLV-III antibody positive man. *Gut* **27**, 587–8.

Kavin H, Jonas RB, Chowdhury L and Kabins S (1986) Acalculous cholecystitis and cytomegalovirus infection in the acquired immunodeficiency syndrome. *Ann. Int. Med.* **104**, 53–4.

Kern P, Toy J and Dietrich M (1985) Preliminary clinical observations with recombinant interleukin-2 in patients with AIDS or LAS. *Blut* **50**, 1–6.

Kotler DP, Gaetz HP, Lange M, Klein EB and Holt PR (1984) Enteropathy associated with the acquired immunodeficiency syndrome. *Ann. Int. Med.* **101**, 421–8.

Lawrence J (1985) The immune system in AIDS. *Scientific American* **253**, 70–9.

Loveday C and Weller IVD (1987) Care of the antibody-positive patient. In: Pounder RE (ed.) *Advanced Medicine 23,* pp 80–90. London: Royal College of Physicians/Baillière Tindall.

Ma P and Soave R (1983) Three-step stool examination for cryptosporidiosis in ten homosexual men with protracted watery diarrhoea. *J. Infect. Dis.* **147**, 824–8.

Macher AM (1984) Infection in the acquired immunodeficiency syndrome. In: *Acquired Immunodeficiency Syndrome: Epidemiologic, clinical, immunologic, and therapeutic considerations* (Moderator Fauci AS) pp 94–96. *Ann. Int. Med.* **100**, 92–100.

Margulis SJ, Honig CL, Soave R et al (1986) Biliary tract obstruction in the acquired immunodeficiency syndrome. *Ann. Int. Med.* **105**, 207–10.

Mindel A, Weller IVD, Faherty A et al (1984) Prophylactic oral acyclovir in recurrent genital herpes. *Lancet* **ii**, 57–9.

Modigliani R, Bories C, Charpentier Y Le et al (1985) Diarrhoea and malabsorption in acquired immune deficiency syndrome: a study of four cases with special emphasis on opportunistic protozoan infestations. *Gut* **26**, 179–87.

Nadelman RB, Mathur-Wagh U, Vancovitz SR and Mildvan D (1985) Salmonella bacteremia associated with the acquired immunodeficiency syndrome (AIDS). *Arch. Intern. Med.* **145(11)**, 1968–71.

Nime FA, Barek JD, Page DC, Holscher MA and Yardley JH (1976) Acute enterocolitis in a human being infected with the protozoan cryptosporidium. *Gastroenterology* **70**, 592–8.

Orenstein MS, Tavitian A, Yonk B et al (1985) Granulomatous involvement of the liver in patients with AIDS. *Gut* **26**, 1220–5.

Portnoy D, Whiteside ME, Buckley III E and MacLeod CL (1984) Treatment of Intestinal cryptosporidiosis with Spiramycin. *Ann. Int. Med.* **101**, 202–4.

Rashleigh-Belcher HJC, Carne CA, Weller IVD, Smith AM and Russell RCG (1986) Surgical biopsy for persistent generalised lymphadenopathy. *Br. J. Surg.* **73**, 183–5.

Richman DD, Fischl MA, Grieco MH et al (1987) The toxicity of azidothymidine (AZT) in the treatment of patients with AIDS and AIDS-related complex. *N. Eng. J. Med.* **317**, 192–7.

Rotterdam H and Sommers SC (1985) Alimentary tract biopsy lesions in the acquired immune deficiency syndrome. *Pathology* **17(2)**, 181–92.

Safai B and Weiss H (1984) Clinical manifestations of Kaposi's sarcoma. In Ma P and Armstrong D (eds) *AIDS and Infections of Homosexual Men*, Chap. 16, pp 211–214. New York: Yorke Medical Books.

Sivak SL and Wormser GP (1985) How common is HTLV-III infection in the United States? *N. Eng. J. Med.* **313**, 1352.

Sloper KS, Dourmashkin RR, Bird RB, Slavin G and Webster ADB (1982) Chronic malabsorption due to cryptosporidiosis in a child with immunoglobulin deficiency. *Gut* **23**, 80–2.

Soave R, Danner RL, Honig CL et al (1984) Cryptosporidiosis in homosexual men. *Ann. Int. Med.* **100**, 504–11.

Volberding P, Conant MA, Stricker RB and Lewis BJ (1983) Chemotherapy in advanced Kaposi's sarcoma. *Am. J. Med.* **74**, 652–6.

Weber JN, Carmichael DJ, Boylston A et al (1985) Kaposi's sarcoma of the bowel presenting as apparent ulcerative colitis. *Gut* **26**, 295–300.

Weber JN, Clapham PR, Weiss RA et al (1987a) Human immunodeficiency virus infection in two cohorts of homosexual men: neutralising sera and association of anti-gag antibody with prognosis. *Lancet* **i:** 119–22.

Weber JN, Thom S, Barrison I et al (1987b) Cytomegalovirus colitis and oesophageal ulceration in the context of AIDS: clinical manifestations and preliminary report of treatment with Foscarnet (phosphonoformate). *Gut* **28,** 482–7.

Weiss RA, Clapham RP, Cheingsong-Popov R et al (1985) Neutralising antibodies to human T-lymphotropic virus type III. *Nature* **316,** 69–71.

Weller IVD (1985) The gay bowel. *Gut* **26,** 869–75.

Weller IVD (1986) Gay gastroenterology. In Pounder RE (ed.) *Recent Advances in Gastroenterology 6,* London: Churchill Livingstone, pp 161–80.

Wong-Staal F and Gallow RC (1985) Human T-lymphotropic retroviruses. *Nature* **317,** 393–403.

Ziegler JL, Beckstead JH, Volberding P et al (1984) Non-Hodgkin's lymphoma in 90 homosexual men: relation to generalised lymphodenopathy and the acquired immunodeficiency syndrome. *N. Engl. J. Med.* **311,** 565–70.

Key Developments in Gastroenterology
Edited by P. R. Salmon
© 1988 John Wiley & Sons Ltd

7

Recent Advances in Imaging the Jaundiced Patient

W. R. Lees

The Middlesex Hospital, London

Diagnostic Radiology

Present status of non-invasive imaging

It is now universally recognized that ultrasonography is the primary imaging tool in the investigation of jaundice. It is less well recognized that there have been huge advances in ultrasound technology in the past 3–4 years and that in this period progress in CT and cholangiography has been slight.

Modern ultrasound machines are vastly more sophisticated and complex than their predecessors, and digital signal processing is now central to ultrasound development. Synthetic focusing systems now yield a soft tissue resolution of better than 0.5 mm throughout the full depth of the image. Doppler blood flow signals can be obtained from small branches of the portal and hepatic veins and hepatic arteries and have proved valuable in thrombotic processes and chronic liver disease (Figure 1).

The improvements in spatial resolution coupled with new biopsy techniques have brought about an ability to obtain histology from tumours as small as 5–10 mm.

The major criticism levelled at ultrasonography has been its dependence on the operator's skill. These technical developments have largely automated and improved the process of acquisition of images but considerable experience is still needed to unravel the anatomy and pathomorphology of obstructive jaundice.

What the Clinician Should Expect of Ultrasonography in Obstructive Jaundice

Bile duct calibre

The anatomical information given by the ultrasound radiologist should be precise. The calibre of the bile ducts can be measured with an accuracy of 0.5

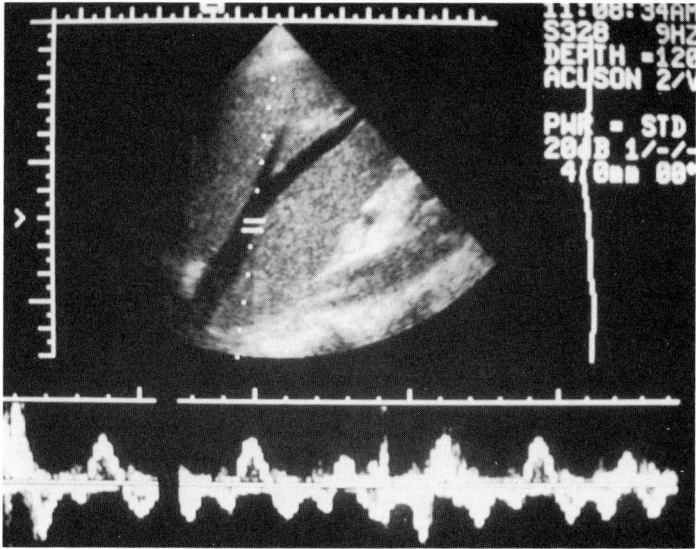

Figure 1. Doppler ultrasound tracings from the left hepatic vein showing blood velocity patterns modulated by retrograde propagation of the right atrial pressure waves. The degree of modulation is affected by the compliance of the surrounding liver tissue.

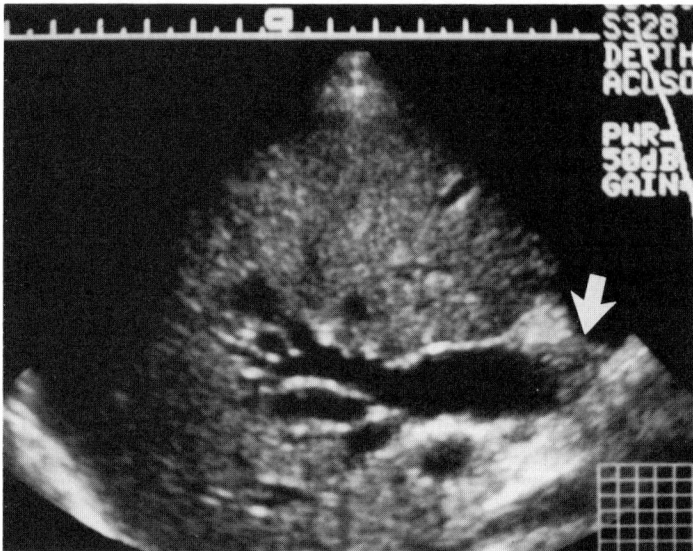

Figure 2. Dilated biliary tree with obstruction from a 1 cm diameter cholangiocarcinoma in the distal CBD (arrowed).

mm. Biliary radicals are not as easily measured as the major ducts but comparison can be made with the associated portal vein; normal bile ducts are 25% of the diameter, 25–50% represents mild dilatation and more than 50% is marked (Figure 2).

Level of obstruction

With modern techniques the termination of the obstructed bile duct can be demonstrated in up to 95% of cases. Borrowing the methods of barium radiology, gas can be displaced from the stomach and duodenum by orally administered fluid and visualisation of the papillary region can be enhanced by duodenal paralysis, and although the papilla cannot always be positively identified the length of the dilated bile duct can be measured from the bifurcation to the obstruction (Figure 3).

Cause of obstruction

The dilated CBD points directly to the obstructing lesion and, provided that the termination is visualised, nearly all tumours and over 75% of gallstones will be positively identified (Laing et al, 1986) (Figure 4).

Of patients with obstructive jaundice, 10 to 20% present as complex problems with multiple disease states. The patient with hepatic cirrhosis and a gallstone at the papilla may show only a minor degree of biliary dilatation. Pancreatic cancer

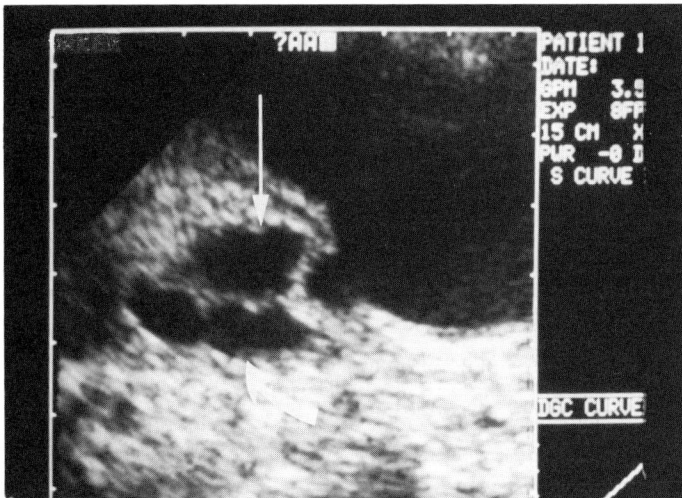

Figure 3. Dilated distal CBD (long arrow) and pancreatic duct (curved arrow) in a patient with an obstructed afferent loop.

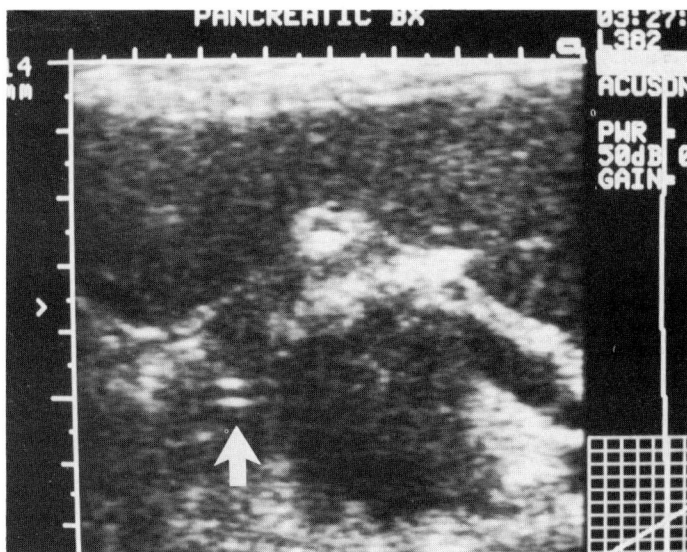

Figure 4. Two centimetre diameter pancreatic carcinoma. A biliary endoprosthesis is present (arrow). Note the eccentric position of the tumour mass in relation to the line of the endoprosthesis.

can induce or co-exist with chronic pancreatitis. Gallstones frequently form above both benign and malignant structures. Cavernous transformation of the portal vein obscures the underlying anatomy, and congenital abnormalities are often more complex than textbook descriptions imply.

Combinations of imaging techniques are usually required to fully resolve these complex diagnostic problems.

Proof of Diagnosis

Invading the obstructed biliary system with a needle or catheter will inevitably contaminate static bile, and progression to multiple liver abscesses and septicaemia can occur in as little as 2–3 weeks if drainage is not established.

In our practice, percutaneous or endoscopic cholangiography is closely followed by biliary drainage usually by endoscopic stent placement, which is successful in over 80% of cases with few complications (Cotton, 1984).

In the past, the failures have been managed by percutaneous placement of a 12–14 French stent but the complication rates are higher than with endoscopic techniques, and this has now been superseded by the combined approach (see below) (Haber and Karten, 1900; Speer et al, 1987).

Once decompression of the biliary tree is achieved, more invasive diagnostic methods can be pursued. Percutaneous cholangiography may be needed to

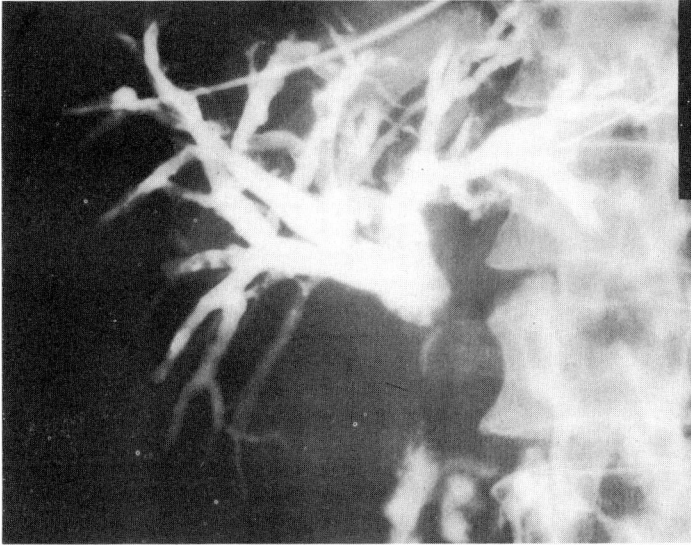

Figure 5. Malignant stricture of the common hepatic duct showing full communication between all intrahepatic biliary radicals.

outline the upper bounds of the stricturing process. Infected bile can be aspirated through a fine needle for culture or tissue fragments can be obtained for cystodiagnosis (Figure 5).

Cytology has not proved as effective for pancreatic and bile duct cancer as it has in other regions, and although the specificity is 100% the sensitivity is no better then 80% and 60% for pancreatic or bile duct cancers respectively (Hall-Craggs and Lees, 1986). Even these poor sensitivities are much better than can be obtained from juice cytology or endoscopic brushings where the yield has never exceeded 20% in our laboratory.

To establish a definite diagnosis by biopsy is important. Even combinations of imaging techniques can fail to provide more than a differential diagnosis.

Histology

In an attempt to improve on these results we have been using an 18 SWG trucut system to gain histological specimens of $1.2 \times 10/20$ mm. This is driven by a mechanical device to rapidly cut the sample (Biopty Tm). This gives great precision, is almost painless and cuts very clean samples from even scirrhous tumours (Figures 6a and 6c). Allied with immunohistochemistry the yield in fibrous biliary and pancreatic cancers has improved significantly and tumour typing is now possible (Lees et al, 1986) (Figure 7). If the biliary tree is decompressed, significant leakage does not occur. We have experienced only two

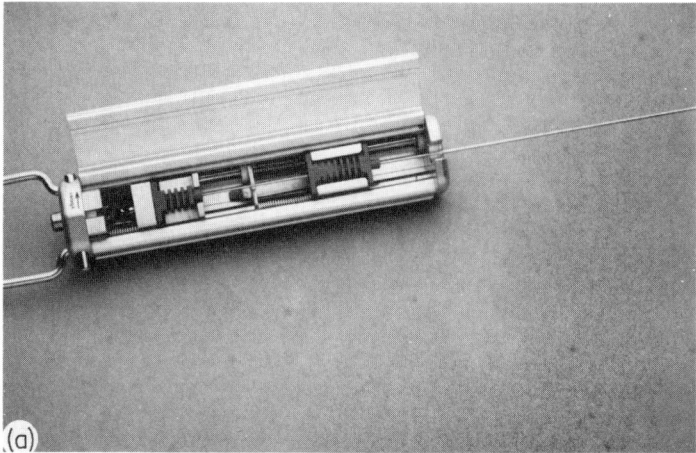

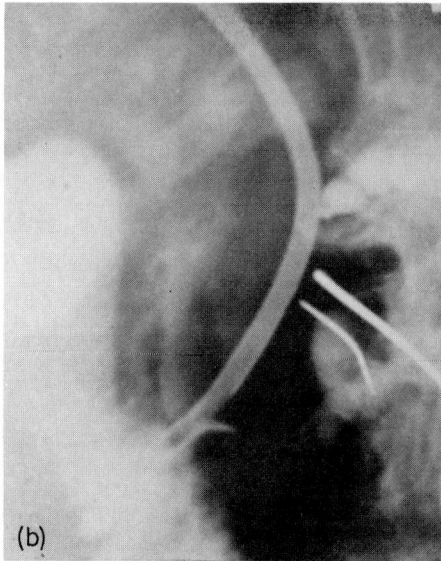

Figure 6. (a) Biopsy device loaded with an 18-gauge trucut needle, cocked and ready to fire. (b) Percutaneous 18-gauge trucut biopsy of a malignant stricture of the common bile duct. The biliary tree has been decompressed by an endoprosthesis and the main pancreatic duct has been outlined by contrast introduced percutaneously by ultrasound guided fine needle punctures. Guidance was by a combination of fluoroscopic and ultrasound markers. A 22-gauge needle was inserted alongside the 18-gauge trucut. (c) Pancreatic ductal adenocarcinoma. Following 18-gauge trucut biopsy the tract of the biopsy needle is clearly seen. The specimen obtained can be orientated for the histopathologist precisely in relation to the ultrasound image.

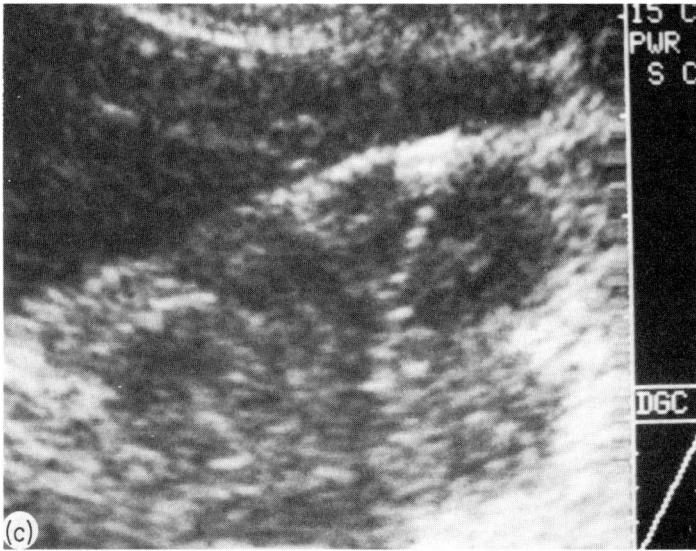

(c)

minor complications in over 70 pancreatic biopsies. In one patient a mild pancreatitis swiftly resolved. In the other a leak of pancreatic juice occurred which required prompt drainage by placement of a percutaneous catheter.

Prospects for Surgery

Our working criteria for resection of pancreatic tumours are:
1) A circumscribed tumour with no evidence of invasion on imaging (Figure 8)
2) Favourable histology
3) No evidence of significant progression at three-month follow-up.
   Conventional cytology is inadequate in separating out that small group of endocrine and other tumours that merit resection (Stark et al, 1981; Teefey et al, 1986).

Staging

Once a specific diagnosis has been achieved, a small percentage of patients will proceed to formal staging using three main methods.
Complete ductography. Full cholangiography and pancreatography to outline strictures in both CBD and pancreatic ducts. If ERCP is incomplete then a percutaneous approach to the two duct system is required.
Dynamic CT scanning is superior to angiography in showing the retroperitoneal extension of the tumour and involvement of the portal veins (Jafri et al, 1984) (Figure 9).

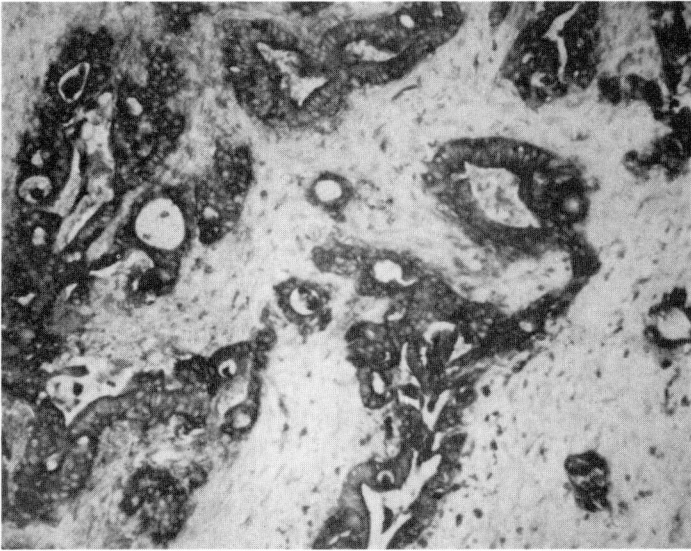

Figure 7. Pancreatic ductal adenocarcinoma stained for CEA expressed
as a surface antigen.

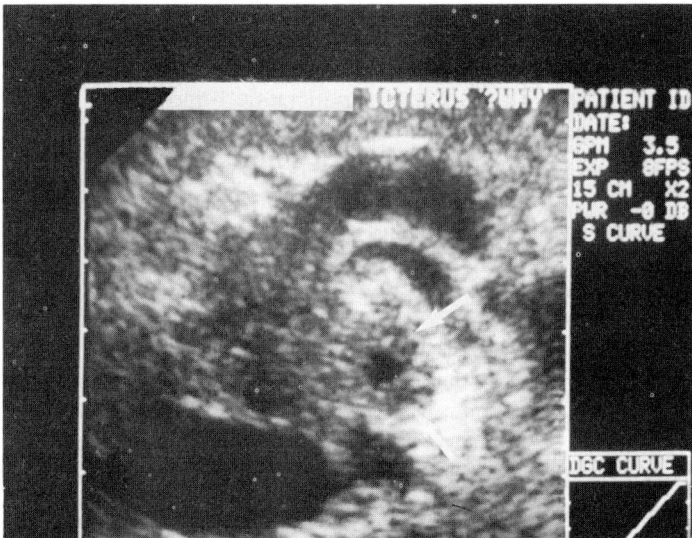

Figure 8. A 25 mm diameter pancreatic carcinoma causing dilatation of
the main pancreatic duct. Invasion of the tumour mass around the origin
of the superior mesenteric artery is clearly demonstrable (arrows).

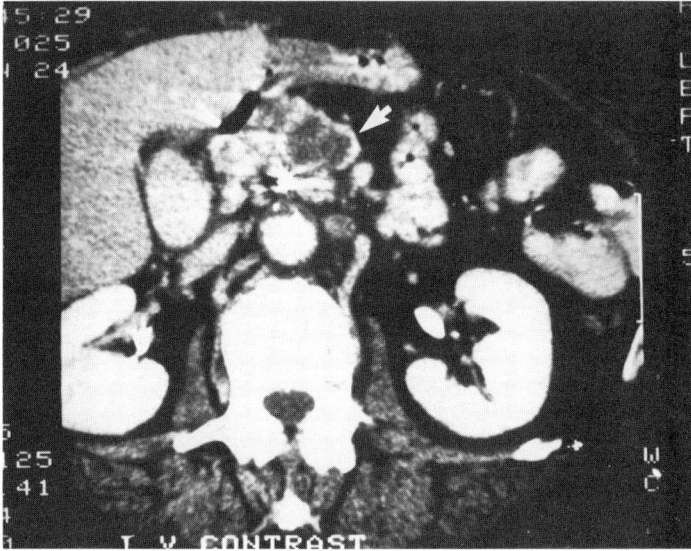

Figure 9. Dynamic contrast enhanced CT scan showing tumour thrombus growing within the portal venous system (arrows).

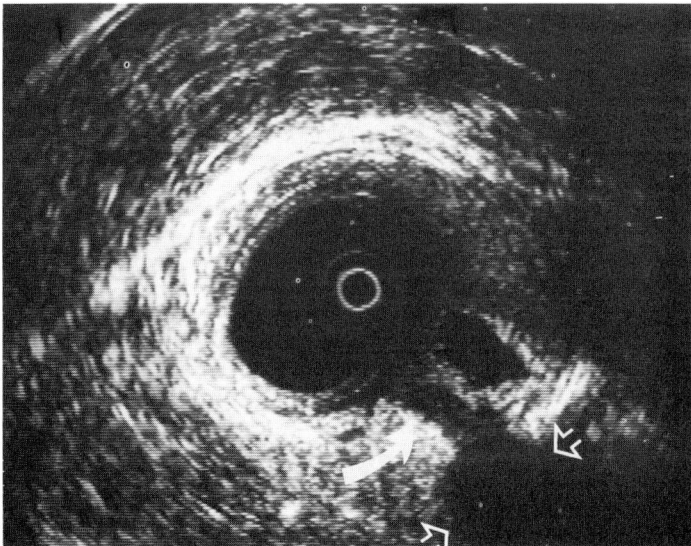

Figure 10. Endoscopic ultrasound of a small carcinoma of the head of the pancreas (arrows) with linear infiltration in the wall of the duodenum and gastric antrum (curved arrows).

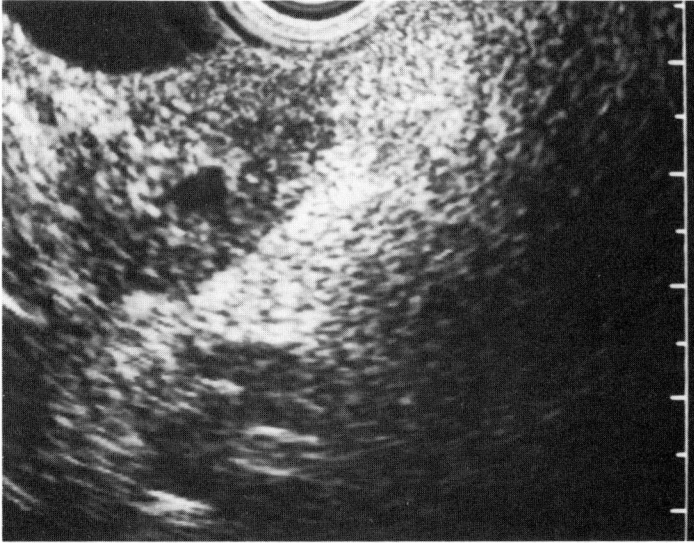

Figure 11. Endoscopic ultrasound of a small tumour of the distal CBD
at its point of occlusion. The narrowed CBD is arrowed. The tumour is
well defined with no evidence of significant invasion in the surrounding
tissues. The tumour was successfully resected.

Endoscopic ultrasonography is a new technique employing a high-frequency high-resolution ultrasound scanner mounted on the tip of a side viewing duodenoscope. This device gives much greater resolution in the region of the head of the pancreas than any other and will show invasion of the walls of the duodenum or portal vein, and involvement of local nodes. The method is simple; the endoscope is placed in the third part of the duodenum and slowly withdrawn around the duodenal loop and along the greater curve of the stomach, scanning the contiguous pancreas all the while. The scan is completed in under 20 minutes and is tolerated as well as any other duodenoscopy.

This technique is now the most precise imaging tool we have for staging pancreatic and bile duct cancer and categorising pancreatic disease (Lees and Rode, 1986) (Figures 10 and 11).

Even though less than 5% of our patients with malignant obstructive jaundice will pass through this presurgical sieve many will already have micrometastases in nodes or liver, and our emphasis is more on favourable histology than favourable morphology.

Surgical planning is greatly enhanced by the use of similar miniature high-frequency ultrasound probes designed for use at laparotomy (Figure 12).

The relationship between diagnostic and therapeutic procedures is given in Figure 13.

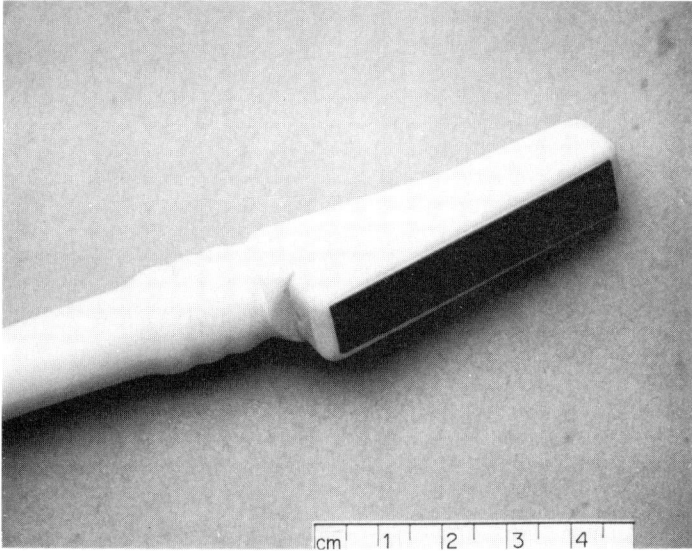

Figure 12. Intraoperative ultrasound probe.

Recent Advances in Therapeutic Radiology

It is not surprising that the complication rates of percutaneous procedures are higher than those of the endoscopy. Liver tissue must be traversed to gain access to the bile ducts and some damage inevitably occurs. The most important factor governing morbidity is the size of the catheter inserted through the liver. Up to 7-8 French, the complication rates are very low. Very large drains not only cause more trauma but often require insertion under general anaesthetic (Hoevels and Ihse, 1979; Mueller et al, 1985; Cooms and Carey, 1983).

The logical solution to the problem is to combine the two methods.

The percutaneous approach to the biliary tree has several advantages:

1) The optimal segment or even branch duct can be punctured under ultrasound control.

2) Initial access to the biliary tree is with a system of less than 1 mm diameter, followed by immediate insertion of a 4 or 5 French working catheter. Only local anaesthesia is required.

3) Radiological guide wire/catheter systems with variable torque control are easier to manipulate through a stricture than the endoscopic equivalents.

4) A guide wire placed through the papilla into the duodenum can be grasped and pulled up the biopsy channel of an endoscope and a 10-12 French diameter stent can then be railroaded up from below sparing the liver from trauma.

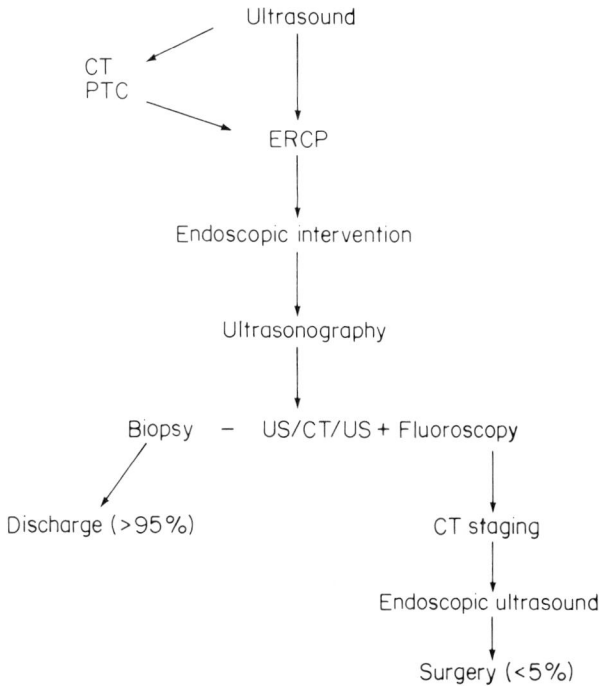

Figure 13. The relationship between diagnostic procedures.

5) Percutaneous drainage can be maintained until endoprosthesis function is
    assured.

This technique has been successful in 68/70 cases where endoscopic
cannulation failed and is increasingly being used as the primary method of
managing high bile duct strictures (Figure 14).

How Much Liver to Drain?

The great success of biliaryendoprosthesis placement in palliating obstructive
jaundice has led to a further problem with high bile duct strictures. How much of
the liver should be drained?

To answer this question we have studied 59 patients with successful
endoscopic stent placement through hilar strictures. The volume of the liver
drained was assessed by two radiologists from cholangiographic and ultrasound
evidence.

Successful palliation was achieved in all patients with more than 10% of the
liver volume drained. Only four infective complications developed in undrained

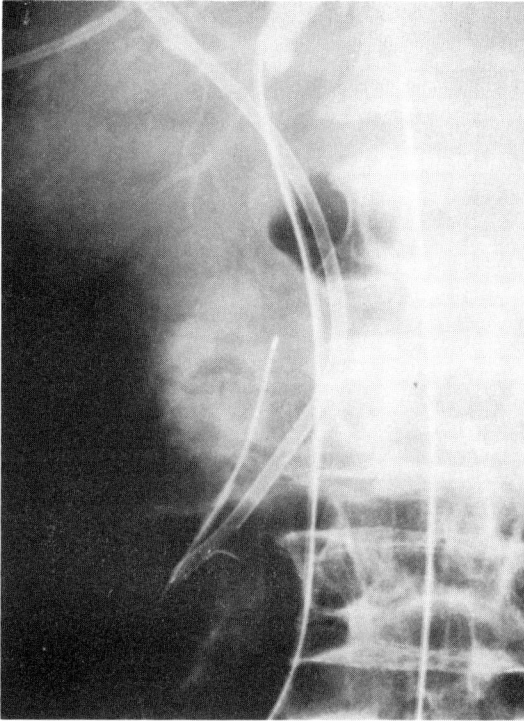

Figure 14. A combined procedure. A long guide wire is seen passing from the left hepatic duct system through a hilar stricture to the duodenum. The right hepatic duct system has already been drained with the same technique and the long endoprosthesis left in situ. A decompressing 5 French percutaneous drain is also seen in situ in the right hepatic duct.

segments, and these were all promptly and successfully treated by further percutaneous drainage into the obstructed segments.

There were nine deaths within 30 days of stent placement (15%). Five died of extensive tumour with less than 15% of the liver drained. Two were in profound hepatorenal failure with 15–30% drainage achieved and one patient with successful 50% drainage died following myocardial infarction.

The message from this study was that striving to gain complete drainage is unnecessary for effective palliation of malignant obstructive jaundice. Patients in hepatorenal failure with tumour deeply invading through the liver do badly and this group would probably benefit from a planned combined procedure, aiming for the largest drainable segment under ultrasound control. This is currently under test (Hall-Craggs et al, 1987).

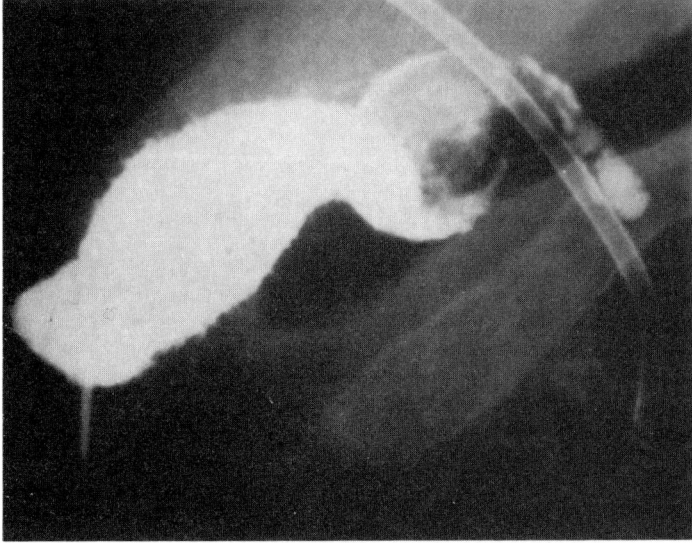

Figure 15. Mirrizi syndrome. The jaundice was relieved by insertion of an endoscopically placed biliary endoprosthesis. Three hundred millilitres of pus were drained from a distended gall bladder via a tube placed under ultrasound guidance. The contrast study displayed was taken several days after successful decompression of both gall bladder and biliary tree. The patient was discharged with a 12 French self-retaining catheter in the gall bladder and after a period of maturation the track was distended to 26 French and access to the gall bladder gained via an operating nephroscope. The stone was disrupted with an electrohydraulic lithotriptor and the fragments removed under direct vision. The patient was discharged within 48 hours of the procedure and the biliary endoprosthesis subsequently removed.

Percutaneous Cholecystostomy

Simple percutaneous drainage of the gall bladder has long been an emergency route for decompression of a low biliary stricture and is now the preferred way of dealing with the infected gall bladder (van Sonnenberg et al, 1986; Hawkins et al, 1985). A simple cholecystostomy can be performed at the time of the initial diagnostic scan under local anaesthesia with immediate benefit. This approach can prove valuable in the more complicated obstructive jaundice, such as the Mirrizi syndrome (Teplick et al, 1982) (Figure 15).

Conclusion

The imaging management of obstructive jaundice continues to be developed and refined; 80% of patients can be diagnosed and decompressed promptly and simply. The remaining 20% need the full range of sophisticated imaging and interventional techniques to establish a complete diagnosis.

References

Cooms HG and Carey PH (1983) Large-bore, long biliary endoprostheses (biliary stents) for improved drainage. *Radiology* **148**, 89–94.

Cotton PB (1984) Endoscopic methods for relief of malignant obstructive jaundice. *World J. Surg.* **8**, 854–61.

Haber GB and Karten PP (1900) Complications of endobiliary prostheses. *Gastrointest. Endosc.* **31**, A168.

Hall-Craggs MA and Lees WR (1986) Fine-needle aspiration biopsy: pancreatic and biliary tumours. *AJR* **147**, 399.

Hall-Craggs MA, Speer T and Lees WR (1987) Drainage of high biliary strictures: single or multiple endoprostheses? (in press).

Hawkins IF Jr (1985) Percutaneous cholecystostomy. *Semin. Interven. Radiol.* **2**, 97.

Hoevels J and Ihse I (1979) Percutaneous transhepatic insertion of a permanent endoprosthesis in obstructive lesions of the extrahepatic bile ducts. *Gastrointest. Radiol.* **4**, 367–77.

Jafri SZH, Aizen AM, Glazer GM et al (1984) Comparison of CT and angiography in assessing resectability of pancreatic carcinoma. *AJR* **142**, 525.

Laing FC, Jeffrey RB Jr, Wing VW and Nyberg DA (1986) Biliary dilatation: defining the level and case by real-time US. *Radiology* **160**, 846.

Lees WR and Rode J (1986) 18 swg cutting biopsy of the pancreas: feasibility, results and safety. *Radiology* 161 (P) Special Edition. RSNA Scientific Program p 347.

Lees WR, Frost R, Shorvon PJ and Cotton PB (1986) Pancreatic endosonography. *Radiology* 161 (P) Special Edition. RSNA Scientific Program p 329.

Mueller PR, Ferrucci JT, Teplick SK et al (1985) Biliary stent endoprostheses: analysis of complications in 113 patients. *Radiology* **156**, 637–9.

Speer AG, Cotton PB, Russell RCG et al (1987) Endoscopic or percutaneous stents for poor risk patients with malignant obstructive jaundice: a prospective randomised trial (in press).

Stark DD, Moss AA, Goldberg HI and Derong CW (1981) CT of pancreatic islet cell tumours. *Radiology* **150**, 491.

Teefey SA, Stephens DH and Steedy PF (1986) CT appearance of primary pancreatic lymphoma. *Gastrointest. Radiol.* **11**, 41.

Teplick SK, Wolferth CC Jr, Hayes MF Jr and Amrom G (1982) Percutaneous cholecystostomy in obstructive jaundice. *Gastrointest. Radiol.* **7**, 259.

van Sonnenberg E, Wittich GR, Casola G et al (1986) Diagnostic and therapeutic percutaneous gallbladder procedures. *Radiology* **160**, 23.

Key Developments in Gastroenterology
Edited by P. R. Salmon
© 1988 John Wiley & Sons Ltd

8

Surgical Aspects of Acute Pancreatitis

R. C. N. Williamson

Bristol Royal Infirmary, Bristol

Introduction

Although acute pancreatitis has been recognised as a common abdominal emergency for many years, it remains a mysterious and challenging disease. There are some clearcut predisposing causes, notably gallstones, alcoholism and occasionally cannulation or incision of the pancreatic papilla; yet the pathogenesis of the disease is ill understood. We do not have the answers to several crucial questions. Is duodenopancreatic reflux, papillary obstruction or pancreatic hypersecretion the predominant mechanism leading to acinar rupture and release of activated enzymes within the parenchyma of the gland? Does oedematous pancreatitis always precede haemorrhagic pancreatitis, for if so timely therapy might interrupt the process? Do gallstone pancreatitis and alcoholic pancreatitis have a common pathogenesis? Indeed, is there such an entity as acute alcoholic pancreatitis, or do attacks of pain and hyperamylasaemia in an alcoholic always imply pre-existing structural damage to the gland? In other words is the term 'acute-on-chronic pancreatitis' semantic-ally preferable for the attacks that befall those who chronically abuse alcohol?

When the causation of the disease is so obscure, it is little wonder that treatment remains empirical. Early death often occurs from hypovolaemic shock, especially in the elderly with compromised cardiopulmonary function who tolerate poorly substantial fluid shifts; a close correlation exists between the age of the patient and the risk of death (Figure 1). With the possible exception of nasogastric intubation, accurate intravenous replacement of fluid, electrolyte and protein loss is the one therapy that is universally accepted. Almost all the specific treatments that have been tried have failed to show a definite advantage when properly put to the test. Several of these treatments have had a plausible theoretical basis, but all too frequently they have been discarded as initial optimism gives way to a more rational assessment. In few other causes of the acute abdomen are therapeutic options so uncertain and the need for controlled prospective trials so important.

1968-79

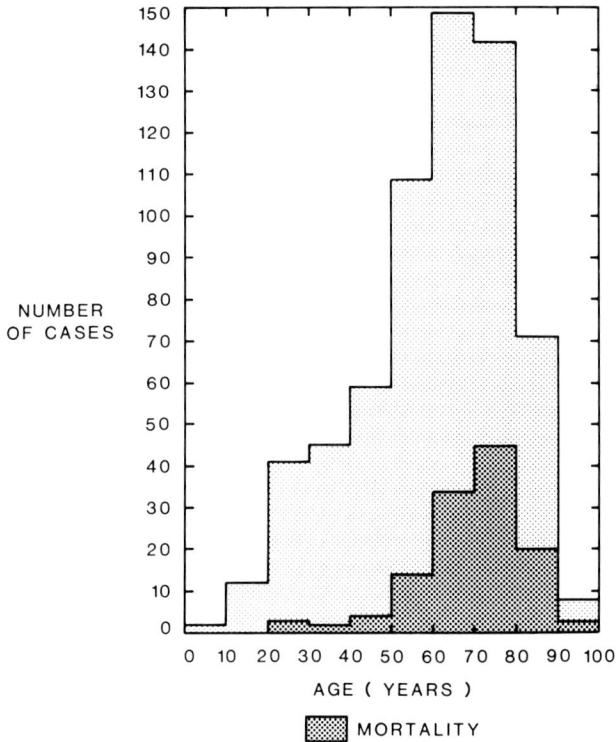

Figure 1. Incidence and mortality rate of acute pancreatitis (first attack) as related to age (Corfield et al, 1985a). Reprinted from *Gut* by kind permission of the publishers.

Since acute pancreatitis nearly always presents with abdominal pain and peritonitis, admission to a surgical ward is the rule in Britain. Probably the only exception is when patients with circulatory collapse are thought to have sustained a cardiac or respiratory disaster. A surgical ward is the correct destination in my opinion, partly because of the risk of missing other abdominal emergencies that need urgent operation. Moreover, a proportion of patients with severe attacks of pancreatitis will develop one or more serious complications that require laparotomy. However, the role of operations in the management of acute pancreatitis is no less controversial than other aspects of the disease. This review presents a brief profile of acute pancreatitis, considers the prediction of severity and then focusses on the role of the surgeon in this disease.

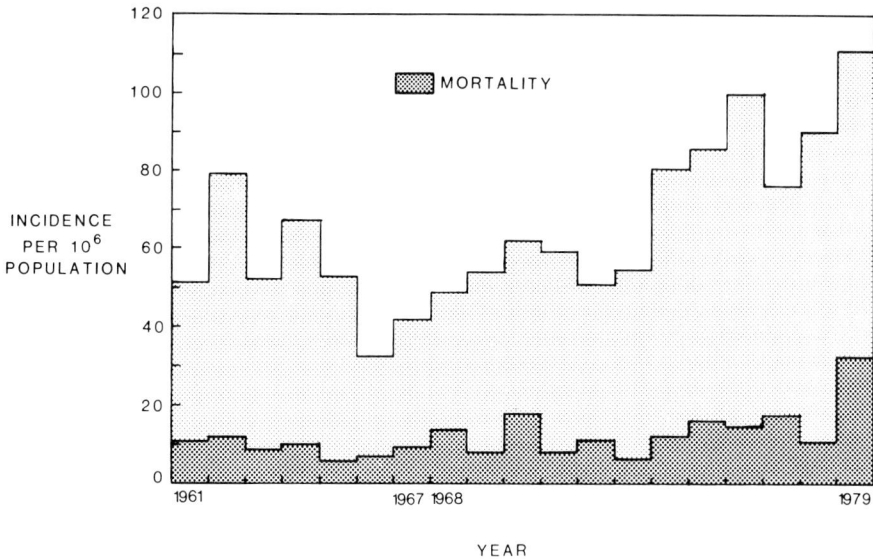

Figure 2. Annual incidence and mortality rate of acute pancreatitis (first attack) in Bristol between 1968 and 1979 (Corfield et al, 1985a). Reprinted from *Gut* by kind permission of the publishers.

Profile of Acute Pancreatitis

Incidence

The natural history of acute pancreatitis has been documented over a 30-year period in Bristol, initially by Trapnell (1950–1967) and latterly by ourselves (1968–1979) (Trapnell and Duncan, 1975; Corfield et al, 1985a). A catchment population of about 800 000 is served by three hospitals in the city with general surgical beds: Bristol Royal Infirmary, Southmead and Frenchay Hospitals. Altogether the case records of 1240 patients have been studied. The data reveal a stepwise increase in the annual incidence of the disease from about 50 cases per million population at first to approximately double this figure by the late 1970s (Figure 2). These figures refer to first attacks of acute pancreatitis, which outnumber recurrent attacks by at least six to one (Corfield et al, 1985a). In Nottingham there was an annual incidence of 48 cases per million during the years 1969–1976 (Bourke et al, 1979), while in Birmingham the incidence steadily increased between 1967 and 1980 (De Bolla and Obeid, 1984).

Part of the apparent increase in diagnosing acute pancreatitis could be due to better recognition of the disease and a greater inclination to measure serum amylase in patients admitted with an unexplained acute abdomen; certainly local interest in the disease has remained high as a result of consecutive studies. Were this the sole explanation, however, the number of patients with a severe attack would be 'diluted' by those with mild disease (requiring a high index of suspicion for diagnosis). To the contrary, our statistics reveal that the proportion of fatal cases has remained about the same between 1950 and 1980, and the Birmingham figures (1967–1980) tell the same story (De Bolla and Obeid, 1984). We therefore believe that there has been a genuine increase in the incidence of acute pancreatitis.

Diagnosis

Our criteria for diagnosing acute pancreatitis are first a consistent clinical picture, including epigastric and back pain (usually of rapid onset), vomiting, peritonitis (epigastric or generalised) and variable degrees of shock, dyspnoea and cyanosis. These features are coupled with a serum amylase level in excess of 1000 Somogyi units per 100 ml (normal < 160), which roughly corresponds in our laboratory to 2000 IU/l as measured by the Phadebas kit (normal < 300) (Corfield et al, 1985a). Plain abdominal radiographs are obtained to help exclude mimicking conditions, such as perforated peptic ulcer and small bowel obstruction or infarction. Leucocytosis is frequently present.

The critical level of hyperamylasaemia regarded as pathognomonic of acute pancreatitis is a matter of controversy. It is generally higher in the UK than the USA (Williamson, 1984). We chose a relatively high level to conform with Trapnell's previous study, thus minimising the risk of false positive values but doubtless missing a certain number of milder attacks of pancreatitis. In practice, 10% of that attacks of acute pancreatitis in our retrospective series ($n = 737$) were first diagnosed at laparotomy and another 6% at autopsy, although not all of these patients had had an amylase estimation (Corfield et al, 1985a). Overall, the serum amylase was misleadingly low (false negative) in 6.5% of patients tested. In tune with other British authors (Imrie and Shearer, 1986; Mayer et al, 1984) we now accept a serum amylase value above 1200 IU/l (600 Somogyi units/100 ml) as diagnostic of acute pancreatitis.

Diagnosis may be refined by measuring serum isoenzymes of amylase and urinary amylase, although the value of the amylase/creatinine clearance ratio has yet to be established (Imrie and Shearer, 1986; Williamson, 1984). Several other pancreatic enzymes can be detected in increased concentration in the serum or urine. Of these, trypsin is specific to the pancreas and serum levels may remain elevated for longer than those of lipase, phospholipase or catalase (Berry et al, 1982). However, serum lipase can be measured more simply nowadays and may be useful in clinching the diagnosis when the amylase is equivocal (Imrie and Shearer, 1986). Although the total amylase content in the blood remains the yardstick in routine clinical practice (Bouchier, 1985), it is generally accepted that the degree of elevation does not correlate with the severity of the attack (Williamson, 1984).

Table 1. Aetological causes of acute pancreatitis in Bristol

	First attacks ($n = 638$)		Recurrent attacks ($n = 99$)	
	Cases (%)	Deaths (%)	Cases (%)	Deaths (%)
Gallstones	50	33	51	33
Alcoholism	8	6	14	0
Idiopathic	23	23	29	42
Postoperative	3	9	0	0
Neoplasia	2	7	0	0
Miscellaneous	7	15	4	8
Unknown	7	7	2	17

From Corfield et al (1985a).

Aetiology

Upwards of half the patients in Bristol with acute pancreatitis have concomitant gallstones (Table 1) (Corfield et al, 1985b). No doubt the association is underplayed in retrospective series, since some patients are inadequately investigated or documented for various reasons. In Bristol the incidence was around 50% throughout the 30-year period reviewed (Trapnell and Duncan, 1975; Corfield et al, 1985a), but in a small prospective series it rose to 64% when patients were more intensively studied (Cooper et al, 1982). Small gallstones are usually to blame (Figure 3) (Armstrong et al, 1985), and these can be easy to miss

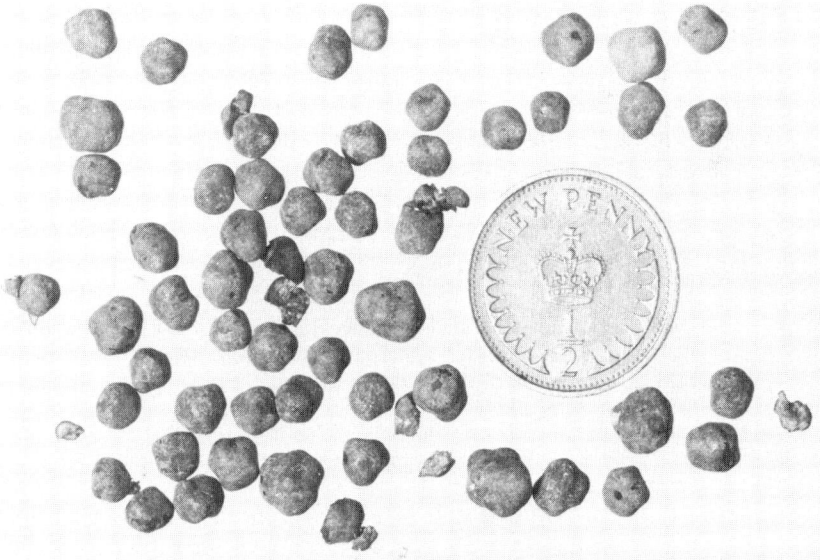

Figure 3. Gallstones contained in the gallbladder removed from a 20-year-old woman 12 days after an attack of acute pancreatitis. Multiple small calculi are typical of acute pancreatitis.

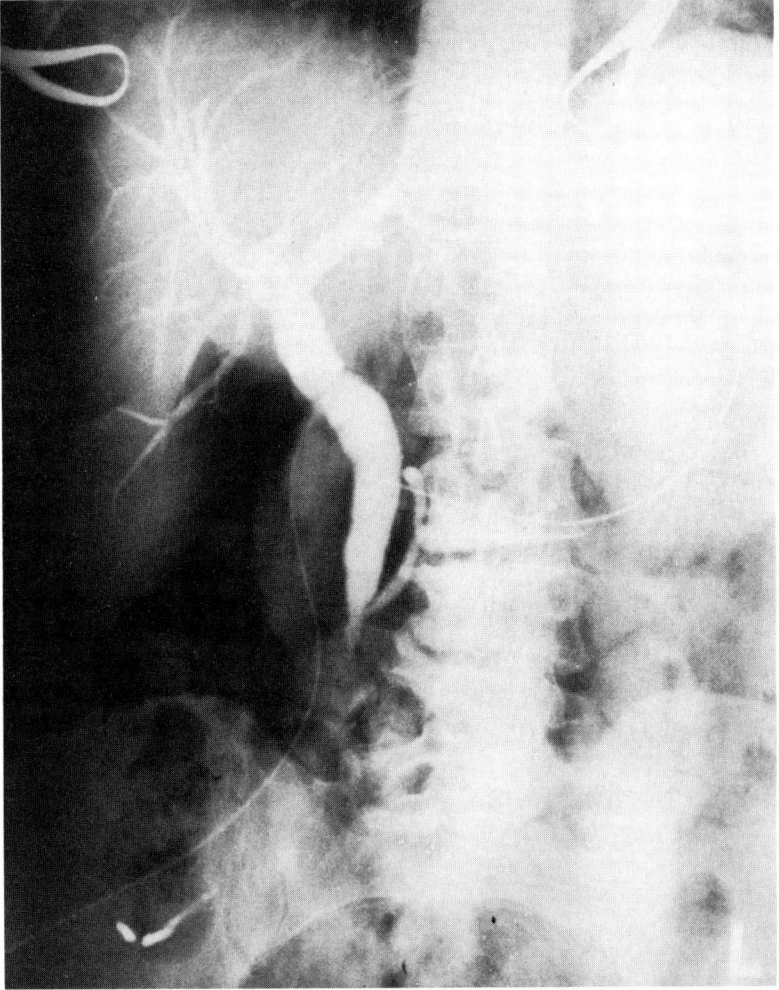

Figure 4. Peroperative cholangiogram of a woman of 71 years who was explored 24 hours after the onset of symptoms of acute pancreatitis. A gallbladder containing several small calculi was removed. The cholangiogram shows a dilated bile duct and no passage of contrast to the duodenum, but transduodenal sphincteroplasty showed that the obstruction was only due to oedema of the ampulla; the stone had already passed. Note also reflux of contrast along the major pancreatic duct.

by conventional ultrasonography and cholecystography. There is overwhelming evidence to support the theory that pancreatitis results from migration of one or more calculi down the cystic duct and common bile duct, with temporary impaction in the ampulla of Vater. Thus small stones, a wide cystic duct and the presence of a common channel are frequent accompaniments of acute

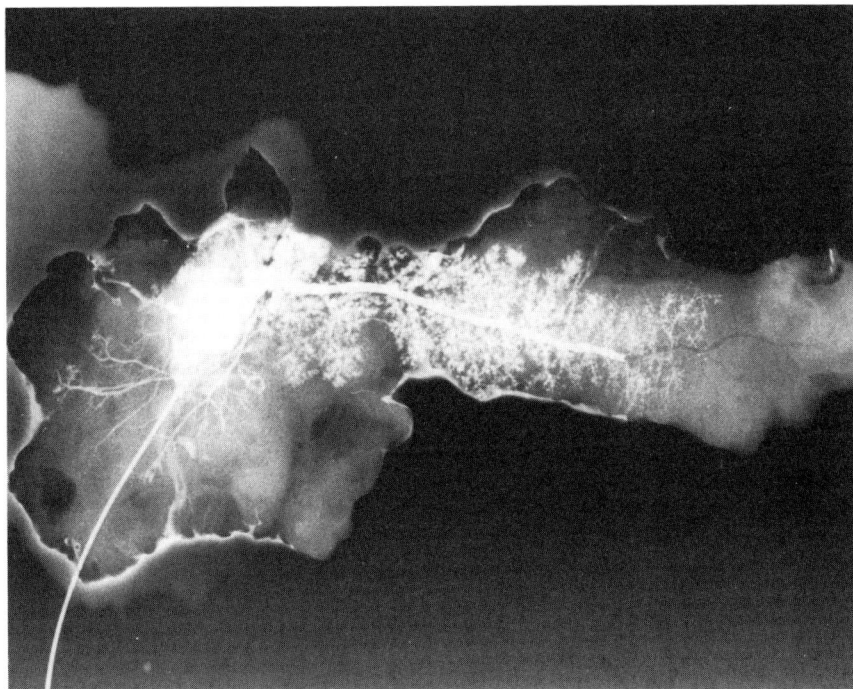

Figure 5. Post-mortem pancreatogram showing an intact ductal tree and relatively normal panenchyme. This patient, a 49-year-old woman, developed fulminating pancreatitis immediately after mitral valve replacement under cardiopulmonary bypass. Laparotomy was performed at 5 days, with radical debridement of a pancreatic abscess and excision of ischaemic transverse colon. Despite peritoneal lavage and a second laparotomy she died at 1 month.

pancreatitis (Kelly, 1984). Stones can usually be found in the common duct if the patient is explored early enough (Armstrong et al, 1985; Stone et al, 1981), or can be retrieved from the faeces during convalescence after an acute attack (Acosta et al, 1977; Kelly, 1980). Lastly, reflux of contrast along the pancreatic duct is often seen during operative cholangiography after an episode of acute pancreatitis (Figure 4).

Alcoholism has steadily increased as a cause of acute pancreatitis in Bristol from 3.7% of first attacks in the 1950s to 10.8% by the end of the 1970s (Corfield et al, 1985a). In Glasgow, a third of patients are alcoholic (Imrie et al, 1978a), in New York City two-thirds (Ranson et al, 1976) and in Atlanta as many as 92% (Satiani and Stone, 1979). The national consumption of alcohol is rising in Britain (James et al, 1974) and possibly in other developed countries.

Postoperative acute pancreatitis is an uncommon but dangerous aetiological variant (Imrie et al, 1978b). In Bristol it contributed 3% of first attacks and 9% of the deaths; half the patients with postoperative pancreatitis died (Corfield et al, 1985a). An accepted complication of surgical or endoscopic procedures on the papilla, acute pancreatitis can occasionally follow almost any type of operation. When it occurs as a complication of cardiopulmonary bypass it is particularly lethal (Figure 5) (Rose et al, 1984).

Acute pancreatitis may develop, often as a terminal event, in patients with varying types of cancer. The tumour is generally a primary or secondary carcinoma of the pancreas itself or adjacent organs. Occasional causes include blunt abdominal trauma, hypothermia, isolated dorsal pancreas (pancreas divisum) and viral infection. Several drugs have been incriminated, often on sketchy criteria. We are not convinced about the aetiological relevance of corticosteroids, nor yet about diabetes and hyperparathyroidism (Corfield et al, 1985a). When all causative factors are taken into account there is still an idiopathic group comprising about 25% of patients, though some of these should strictly be classified as 'unknown' since investigation has been inadequate. A case can be made for investigating all such patients by means of endoscopic retrograde cholangiopancreatography (ERCP), which will diagnose some 'missed' gallstones and the occasional ductal anomaly (Feller, 1984). In fact this investigation is often reserved for patients with recurrent attacks.

Since gallstones are the predominant cause and these are much commoner in women, it is surprising that our sex incidence is almost equal (327:311, female:male). The fact that most alcoholics (90%) were male partly redressed the balance, but no less than 41% of our patients with gallstone pancreatitis were men (Corfield et al, 1985a). Perhaps males are more likely to develop gallstones that migrate, or females have a lower threshold for seeking medical attention and undergoing a prophylactic cholecystectomy.

Outcome

For about three in four patients the course of acute pancreatitis is benign and uncomplicated; the remainder develop serious complications and may die (Cooper et al, 1982; Imrie et al, 1978a; Mayer et al, 1985). Those who survive an early phase of hypovolaemic shock may yet die from sepsis and multiorgan failure. Pancreatic abscess (or necrosis) is a particularly dreaded complication, generally carrying a 30–50% mortality rate (Becker et al, 1984; Shi et al, 1984) though the prognosis may be improving (Warshaw and Jin, 1985). Overall mortality rates in acute pancreatitis vary between 6 and 23% (Renner et al, 1985) and in prospective series they hover around 10% (Williamson, 1984). When pathology records are scrutinised in detail, however, the mortality rate can rise to 20% with the inclusion of moribund patients in whom acute pancreatitis is first diagnosed at autopsy (Corfield et al, 1985a). Indeed, no less than a third of the fatal cases in Bristol belonged to this group of patients. Premortem diagnoses included cardiac or respiratory failure and other causes of peritonitis. In our experience about a third of patients with acute pancreatitis are over the age of 70 years, and symptoms and signs are sometimes difficult to assess in the elderly; they are also more susceptible to complications and death.

If the first attack of pancreatitis continues to convey a substantial risk of death (19.6%), second and subsequent attacks are a little less hazardous though far from innocuous (12.1% died; P<0.08) (Corfield et al, 1985a). This difference is less marked than previously suggested (Trapnell and Duncan, 1975). Alcohol looms larger in the aetiology of recurrent acute pancreatitis than among first attacks, but delayed cholecystectomy is still the major cause (Table 1).

Prediction of Severity

Objectives

When patients are admitted to hospital with acute pancreatitis their initial clinical evaluation will often suggest a severe illness. Yet many of them improve dramatically over the next 1–2 days as a result of fluid replacement and other simple measures. Less often the corollary holds true. The initial appearances are deceptively mild and the patient's condition deteriorates thereafter. The inability of clinical assessment alone to predict the outcome of the disease with any accuracy is established beyond any doubt (Corfield et al, 1985b; McMahon et al, 1980); but it is a major problem in treating pancreatitis.

Early recognition of patients destined to develop serious and perhaps fatal complications would allow them to be followed with much closer scrutiny than might be appropriate for the majority who will quickly recover. After all, intensive care facilities are a limited resource in most hospitals. At present there is no specific treatment that is of proven value in acute pancreatitis. Prospective trials do not support the routine use of glucagon, aprotinin (Trasylol) or peritoneal lavage and have not yet been used to evaluate the role of antibiotics, anticholinergics, fresh frozen plasma, somatostatin, papillotomy or other urgent surgical manoeuvres (Williamson, 1984). Some of these treatments involve extra hazard to patients who are already ill and might well be meddlesome in those with a mild attack of pancreatitis.

We should therefore strive to separate mild and severe attacks as early as possible after the patient is first seen in hospital. However desirable, this remains an elusive goal. The most useful tests are outlined below and considered in greater detail elsewhere (Williamson, 1984).

Individual criteria

The perfect discriminator is simple, safe, quick, cheap, reliable: it is also unavailable. Clinical examination at the outset will only detect a third of severe (i.e. complicated) attacks (Corfield et al, 1985b; McMahon et al, 1980).

Nevertheless, certain physical signs (though often absent) can indicate fulminant pancreatitis. These signs include high fever, marked cyanosis and air hunger, profound shock, tetany, abdominal mass and Grey-Turner's sign (Trapnell, 1966; Jacobs et al, 1977). Likewise hypocalcaemia on admission (<2.0 mmo/l) is specific but insensitive (Cooper et al, 1982); subsequent measurements of serum calcium simply mirror the inevitable fall in serum albumin. Blood gas analysis should be undertaken routinely in acute pancreatitis (Imrie and Shearer, 1986). Besides demonstrating the need for oxygen therapy or even assisted ventilation (Berry et al, 1981), arterial hypoxaemia can be a useful guide to prognosis; a Pao_2 below 8 kPa (60 mmHg) is an unfavourable index (Cooper et al, 1982). However, elderly patients with chest disease may be chronically hypoxaemic.

Several individual criteria have been greeted with enthusiasm yet failed to be taken into routine practice because they are slow to develop, insensitive or unreliable. Circulating levels of methaemalbumin, fibrinogen, complement proteins and endotoxins belong to this group (Williamson, 1984).

Two methods are promising and need further evaluation. Urgent computed tomography (CT) can differentiate between oedematous (mild) and haemorrhagic (severe) pancreatitis (Dammann et al, 1980; Hill et al, 1982); there are obvious logistic problems in performing this test routinely. Second, the volume and colour of peritoneal fluid obtained by paracentesis can be invaluable in identifying a severe attack (Pickford et al, 1977). This is clearly an invasive procedure, and we had 2 cases of visceral puncture among 252 patients tested (0.8%) (Corfield et al, 1985b). Bladder injury in one of these would have been avoided if the protocol had been respected and urethral catheterisation performed before insertion of the peritoneal dialysis catheter. The other patient had a midline subumbilical scar, and a catheter correctly inserted in the right iliac fossa entered the caecum. Following recognition and repair of the injury recovery was uneventful. Abdominal paracentesis does have two important advantages as a predictor of severity. It gives an answer more quickly than any other technique and occasionally it corrects an erroneous diagnosis of acute pancreatitis, when pure blood, bile or gastric juice are retrieved from the peritoneal cavity.

Scoring systems

By careful analysis of retrospective data Ranson identified 11 factors that correlated with severity (Ranson et al, 1974). When three or more were positive, over 90% of patients went on to develop serious complications or death in a prospective study of 200 cases (Ranson et al, 1976). These criteria are based on age, leucocytosis, hyperglycaemia, hepatocellular damage, respiratory and renal insufficiency, hypocalcaemia, a falling haematocrit, metabolic acidosis and fluid sequestration. Unfortunately the criteria, which originated from a population of

Table 2 Predictive factors in acute pancreatitis

Age >55 years
White blood cell count $>15 \times 10^9/l$
Blood glucose >10 mmol/l (no diabetic history)
Serum urea > 16 mmol/l (no response to i.v. fluids)
$PaO_2 < 60$ mmHg (<8 kPa)
Serum calcium < 2.0 mmol/l
Serum albumin < 32 g/l
Serum lactic dehydrogenase >600 U /l

Three or more factors = severe disease.
From Blamey et al (1984).

alcoholics, require adjustment for those with gallstone pancreatitis (Ranson, 1979). Imrie encountered the same problem in adapting a similar list of criteria for use in British populations where gallstones predominate (Imrie et al, 1978a; Blamey et al, 1984). His latest selection of multiple laboratory criteria is shown in Table 2.

These scoring systems can be criticised since they are elaborate and it takes up to 48 hours to obtain a complete set of data (Williamson, 1984). Generally by this time the severity of the attack is clinically manifest (McMahon et al, 1980). On the other hand they will give a quick answer in fulminating disease, and the overall Ranson score is useful in assessing the results of different treatment regimens. A prospective study conducted in Bristol, Leeds and Glasgow showed that multiple laboratory criteria had a sensitivity of 61% in predicting a severe attack at a median of 24 hours after admission to hospital (Figure 6) (Corfield et al, 1985b). The sensitivity of abdominal pancreatitis was 53% at a median of 4 hours. Combining the two techniques (together with clinical judgement) gave a sensitivity of 77% overall, rising to 85% in fatal cases and 95% in those dying within 10 days. Thus it is usually feasible to identify the worst cases at an early stage. The remaining sections of this chapter explore the possibility that aggressive therapy is justified in the light of this knowledge.

Operative Management

Diagnostic

There is a group of patients who suffer a rapid onset of epigastric pain, develop signs of diffusing peritonitis and have modest hyperamylasaemia (500–1000 IU/l). They pose a real diagnostic problem. Sometimes the clinical features settle, and a retrospective label of oedematous pancreatitis is applied. At other times alternative diagnoses loom large. Biliary peritonitis, perforated peptic ulcer, gangrenous intestine, high small-bowel obstruction and leaking aortic aneurysm can all lead to an elevated serum amylase. Sometimes abdominal

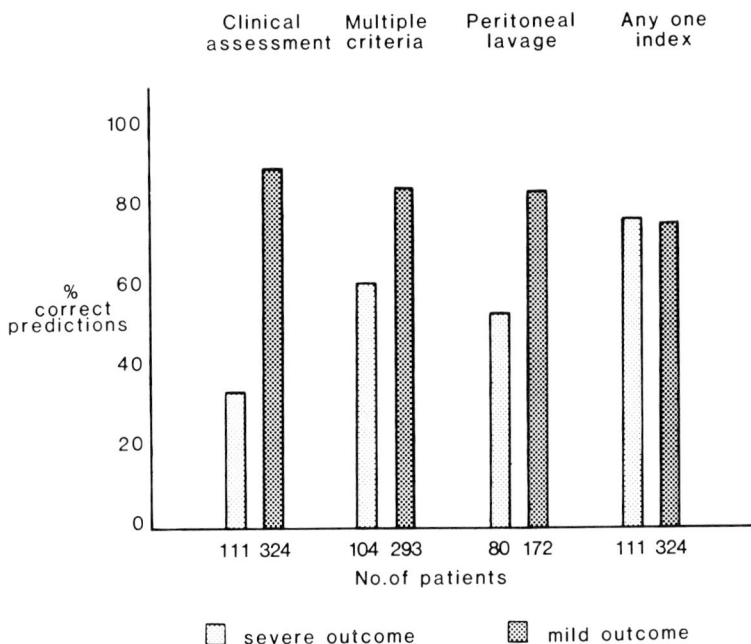

Figure 6. Sensitivity and specificity of three prognostic indices in a prospective study of 435 patients with acute pancreatitis in Bristol, Leeds and Glasgow (Corfield et al, 1985b). Clinical assessment on admission is compared with multiple laboratory criteria and the volume and colour of the peritoneal fluid sampled by paracentesis and lavage. Reprinted by permission of *The Lancet*.

radiographs or paracentesis clarify the diagnosis but if not, the surgeon should proceed to laparotomy without delay. Most mimicking conditions are lethal unless timely operation is performed, whereas diagnostic laparotomy has not been shown to have an adverse effect on the course of an attack of acute pancreatitis (MRC Multicentre Trial, 1977).

What should the surgeon do if he encounters the tell-tale features of acute pancreatitis at laparotomy, namely fat necrosis, retroperitoneal induration and discoloration, and blood-stained ascites? There is no certain answer. My own policy is to deal with gallstones but leave the pancreas alone. Cholecystectomy and operative cholangiography should be performed. A dilated common bile duct should always be decompressed, because ascending cholangitis can precipitate septicaemia and death. Where possible, ductal calculi should be gently removed, including any that are impacted in the ampulla. If necessary transduodenal sphincteroplasty may be undertaken, provided that the surgeon is experienced at this operation and the pancreatitis is relatively mild. Clumsy technique and severe inflammation can lead to duodenal fistula, so that in unfavourable circumstances it is much safer simply to leave a T-tube in the bile duct.

Prophylactic

The most effective way to prevent acute pancreatitis is by performing a timely cholecystectomy. Symptomatic gallstones should be removed in the first place. Following an attack of acute pancreatitis gallstones should be sought in every case; even alcoholics may have cholelithiasis. In women gallstones are especially common as a cause of pancreatitis, and if the ultrasound scan or cholecystogram are in any way equivocal they should be repeated after a short delay. The most certain way of detecting the causative gallstone is to sieve the stools during convalescence (Acosta et al, 1977).

The timing of biliary surgery following an attack of acute pancreatitis has long been a controversial subject; the weight of evidence now suggests that it should be carried out at an early stage, but not urgently (Kelly, 1980; Mayer et al, 1984; Osborne et al, 1981; Ranson, 1979). My own practice is to look hard for gallstones by means of an ultrasound scan within the first few days of the attack and proceed to cholecystectomy during the same admission but after the patient has recovered. Thus operation usually takes place 10–15 days after the onset of symptoms. Complications of cholecystectomy are commoner if operation is performed earlier than this, whereas there is a 32–48% chance of recurrent pancreatitis if gallstone patients are discharged from hospital without cholecystectomy and remain on a waiting list thereafter (Williamson, 1984).

ERCP after an attack of acute pancreatitis may demonstrate ductal changes that could have either predisposed to the attack or resulted from it. Cotton (1980) demonstrated the congenital anomaly of pancreas divisum (isolated dorsal pancreas) in 25% of patients with 'idiopathic' pancreatitis. I have carried out an accessory sphincteroplasty on two such patients but do not believe that the anomaly is a particularly common cause of pancreatitis. Indeed, it might even protect the isolated dorsal pancreas (i.e. the larger moiety) from gallstone pancreatitis. Occasionally ERCP will demonstrate pancreatic ductal ectasia and/or stenosis at the orifice of the duct of Wirsung. Under these circumstances it may be appropriate to improve the drainage of the duct either by double sphincteroplasty or longitudinal pancreaticojejunostomy, depending upon the configuration of the ductal tree.

Hyperparathyroidism was only diagnosed in 2 of the 650 patients we reviewed with acute pancreatitis (Corfield et al, 1985a). When the association is found, however, parathyroidectomy should prevent further attacks. Recently Stone and colleagues (1985) have advocated truncal vagotomy plus Billroth II (Polya) partial gastrectomy for recurrent acute pancreatitis in alcoholics. Both vagal denervation and reduced output of cholecystokinin from the bypassed duodenum might contribute to a lower pancreatic exocrine secretion. Like

McMahon (1986), I am concerned that the disadvantages of gastrectomy might outweigh its advantages in alcoholics who continue to drink.

Therapeutic

Patients who die early from acute pancreatitis sometimes have a gallstone impacted in the ampulla, as Opie showed in 1901. The assumption that continued calculous obstruction of the pancreas underlies the progression of the disease is the basis for Acosta's advocating urgent transduodenal sphincterotomy. By this means he reduced the mortality rate from 16% to 2% and the (additional) morbidity rate from 22% to 15%, using unoperated historical controls for comparison (Acosta et al, 1978). All 46 patients submitted to operation within 48 hours had stones in the bile duct or the stools, and the stone was impacted in 72%. A potentially safer alternative would be urgent endoscopic papillotomy. Several workers have shown that this technique can be safe within the first few days of an attack (Rosseland and Solhaug, 1984; Safrany and Cotton, 1981; Spuy, 1981), but there must be substantial risks in haemorrhagic pancreatitis especially if a 'pre-cut' is required to negotiate the catheter past the stone. In my opinion both these techniques are fraught with hazard in the hands of all but the most skilled practitioners. I have another three caveats:

1) In most countries a sizeable proportion of patients do not have gallstones, and operations on the sphincter might be meddlesome in such cases. The urgent diagnosis of gallstones in acute pancreatitis is a fallible process (Williamson, 1984). Liver function tests are not very discriminating, still less physical signs. Ultrasound and radionuclide scans are often unsatisfactory.

2) Granted the patient has gallstones, the 'criminal calculus' may already have passed (Stone et al, 1981). The patient described in Figure 4 illustrates the point that hold-up of a stone at the papilla can be very transient. Invasive cholangiography, whether transpapillary or transhepatic, could be difficult or dangerous in the early stages of the disease.

3) Granted that the patient has persistent gallstone obstruction, will decompression necessarily abort the pancreatic lesion? I doubt it. I suspect that patients with a fulminant attack may already have inevitable changes in the pancreas, as inflammation, thrombosis and ischaemia continue in a vicious circle. In others with lesser disease prompt disimpaction could well be beneficial, perhaps by preventing bacterial infection of the obstructed pancreas. It is theoretically possible that adequate drainage would necessitate sphincterotomy of the pancreatic duct itself, i.e. operative intervention. To the contrary, Stone describes a gush of pancreatic juice when the ampullary sphincter is divided, i.e. before proceeding to septotomy. Thus, even if the gallstone had already passed (as it often had), dividing the oedematous sphincter was thought to be a valuable manoeuvre (Stone et al, 1981).

Formerly popular, laparotomy to allow decompression of the bile duct and stomach and placement of drains to the pancreatic bed is not of proven benefit (Lawson et al, 1970; Ranson et al, 1974). An addendum to such an operation might be to leave a peritoneal dialysis catheter in the abdomen for subsequent lavage. The catheter can, of course, be inserted percutaneously without the need for operation. Preliminary studies among alcoholic patients in the USA suggested that peritoneal dialysis might improve survival (Ranson and Spencer, 1978; Stone and Fabian, 1980), possibly by removing toxins or vasoactive kinins from the body. Unfortunately our own controlled trial of peritoneal lavage continuing for 72 hours in 91 patients with severe acute pancreatitis showed no advantage whatsoever in terms of morbidity or mortality (Mayer et al, 1985). A crucial factor may have been the long delay (median 38 hours) between onset of symptoms and start of treatment; it is difficult to shorten this interval in ordinary clinical practice. Although hourly irrigation of the abdomen with 2 litres of dialysate was well tolerated in this trial, it did substantially increase protein loss from the body, so the treatment is not innocuous. Another study of peritoneal lavage recently reported from Sweden also shows no benefit in a randomised trial (Ihse et al, 1986).

In patients who are dying of fulminant pancreatitis it is logical to consider total (or subtotal) pancreatectomy, and an early success was reported by Watts in 1963. Sometimes oedema and thrombosis can make for a relatively straightforward resection (Norton and Eiseman, 1974). However, the overall mortality rate is formidable, being at least one-third and often very much higher (Kivilaasko et al, 1981; Ranson et al, 1974; Smadja and Bismuth, 1984). The main problems are haemorrhage, either at the time or later, and continuing sepsis. Moreover, in alcoholics at least, the survivors of these heroic operations can have persistent problems with diabetes and polyneuropathy (Nordback and Auvinen, 1985). I am not enthusiastic about major resectional procedures undertaken within a few days of the start of an attack of acute pancreatitis. I accept that a truly necrotic pancreas should be removed, if necessary piecemeal. My own experience suggests that all too often the pancreas remains alive and active (Figure 5) and that the necrosis is confined to the fat and other retroperitoneal tissues. Histological examination of resection specimens has shown that 'necrotic' pancreas is indeed often still viable (Nordback et al, 1985). It remains to be seen whether serial CT scans will identify a group of patients in whom pancreatectomy might be appropriate, though the operation can never be safe.

For complications

The 'surgical' complications of acute pancreatitis are chiefly pseudocyst and abscess, with or without pancreatic necrosis and haemorrhage. Occasional indications for operation are duodenal obstruction requiring gastroenterostomy,

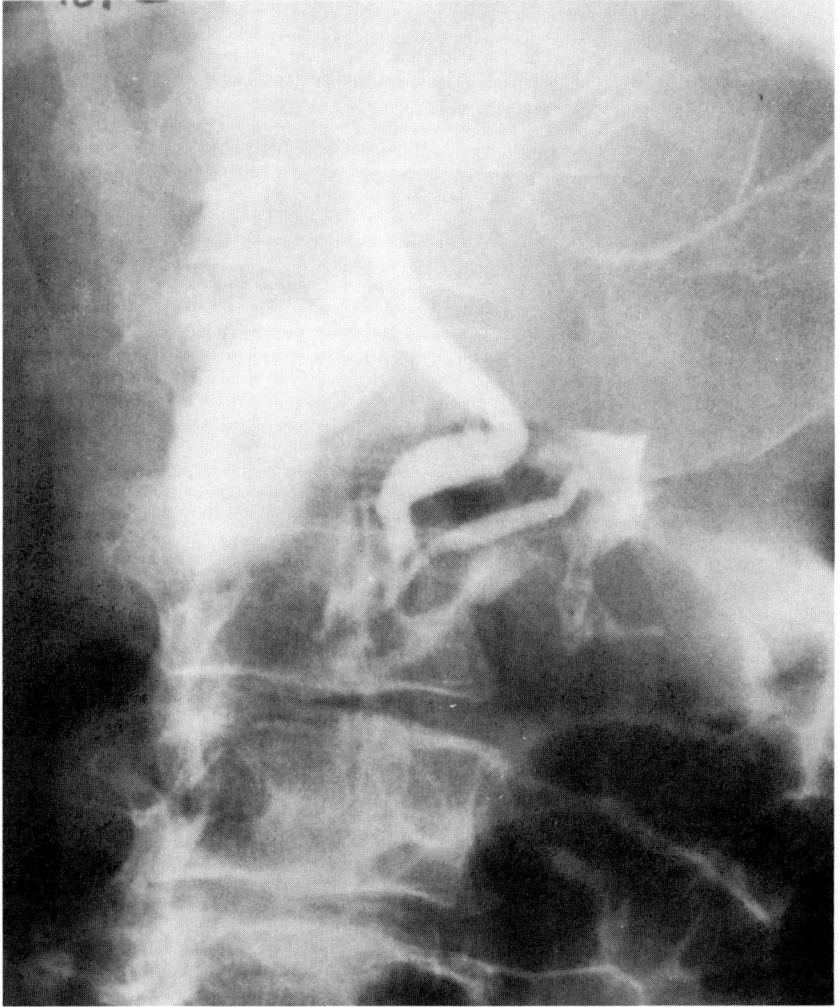

Figure 7. ERCP in a man of 68 years with a pancreatic fistula two months after external drainage of a pancreatic abscess. The pancreatogram shows spillage of contrast from the duct in the pancreatic neck. The fistula closed spontaneously 2–3 weeks later. Note the tell-tale calculus in the gallbladder. Subsequent cholecystectomy was safely undertaken.

colonic infarction and persisting pancreatic fistula after drainage of an abscess. Most fistulas close spontaneously, however (Figure 7). The middle colic vessels may undergo thrombosis when they become involved by direct extension of a necrotising peripancreatitis, in which case resection of the transverse colon or entire right colon should be followed by exteriorisation of the bowel (Figure 5) (Schein et al, 1985).

A pancreatic pseudocyst is a loculated effusion, rich in amylase, which develops within the vicinity of the pancreas within 1–2 weeks of the acute attack. It will often produce a palpable mass and renewed elevation of serum amylase, though there are occasional diagnostic pitfalls (Figure 8) (Gillatt et al, 1986). The cyst is usually found in the lesser sac but sometimes in front of the gland, between the leaves of the greater or lesser omentum, or further afield beneath the diaphragm or within the chest. The increasing use of ultrasonography and CT scan (Figure 9) has shown that these effusions develop quite frequently after an attack of acute pancreatitis. Although pseudocysts are more common in alcoholic than gallstone pancreatitis (15% v 3%), haemorrhage and sepsis are more likely to complicate cysts associated with gallstones (Imrie and Shearer, 1986). Many small cysts subside spontaneously (O'Malley et al, 1985), but others expand and cause symptoms by compressing the stomach (Figure 9) or bile duct. Cysts can be aspirated percutaneously, but recurrence is likely to necessitate repeated aspiration (Colhoun et al, 1984). They can even be drained by an endoscopic approach, using a modified papillotome (Kozarek et al, 1985), or by percutaneous cystgastrostomy under CT control (Bernardino and Amerson,

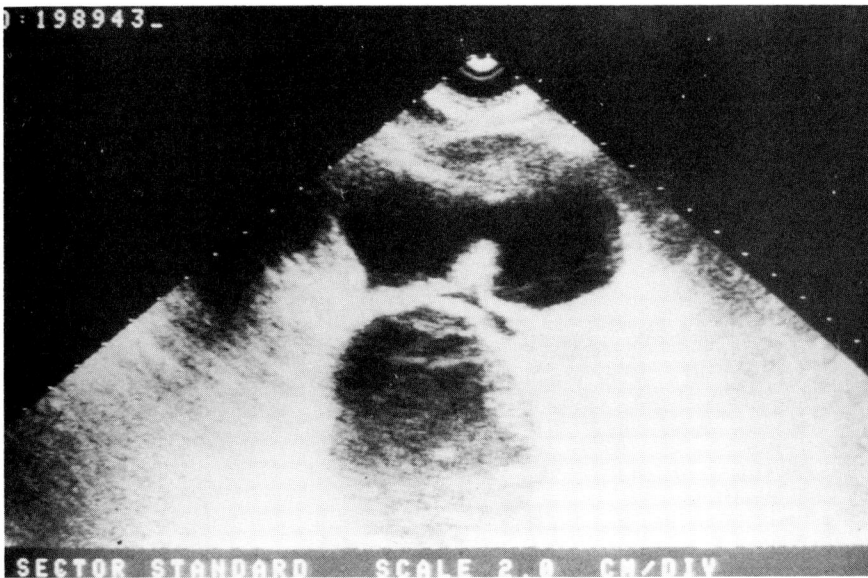

Figure 8. Ultrasound scan of the upper abdomen showing a transonic mass in the region of the lesser sac. The patient was a woman of 56 years who presented with severe pain, a tender epigastric mass and a serum amylase of 4870 IU/l. She was thought to have acute pancreatitis and a pseudocyst but at laparotomy was found to have gross distension of the afferent loop associated with previous Polya gastrectomy (Gillatt et al, 1986). Reprinted from *Pancreas* by kind permission of the Editor.

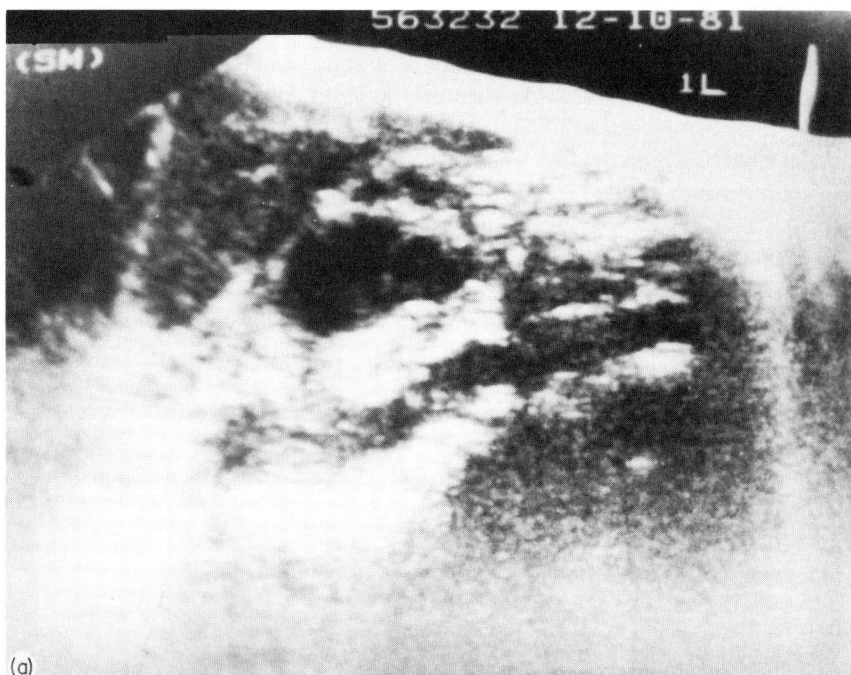

(a)

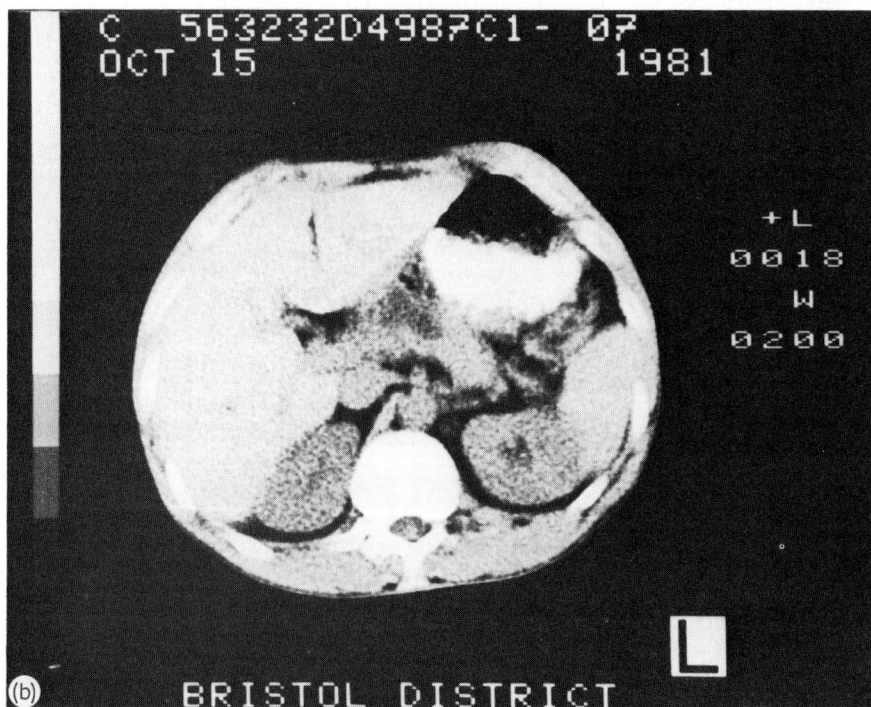

(b)

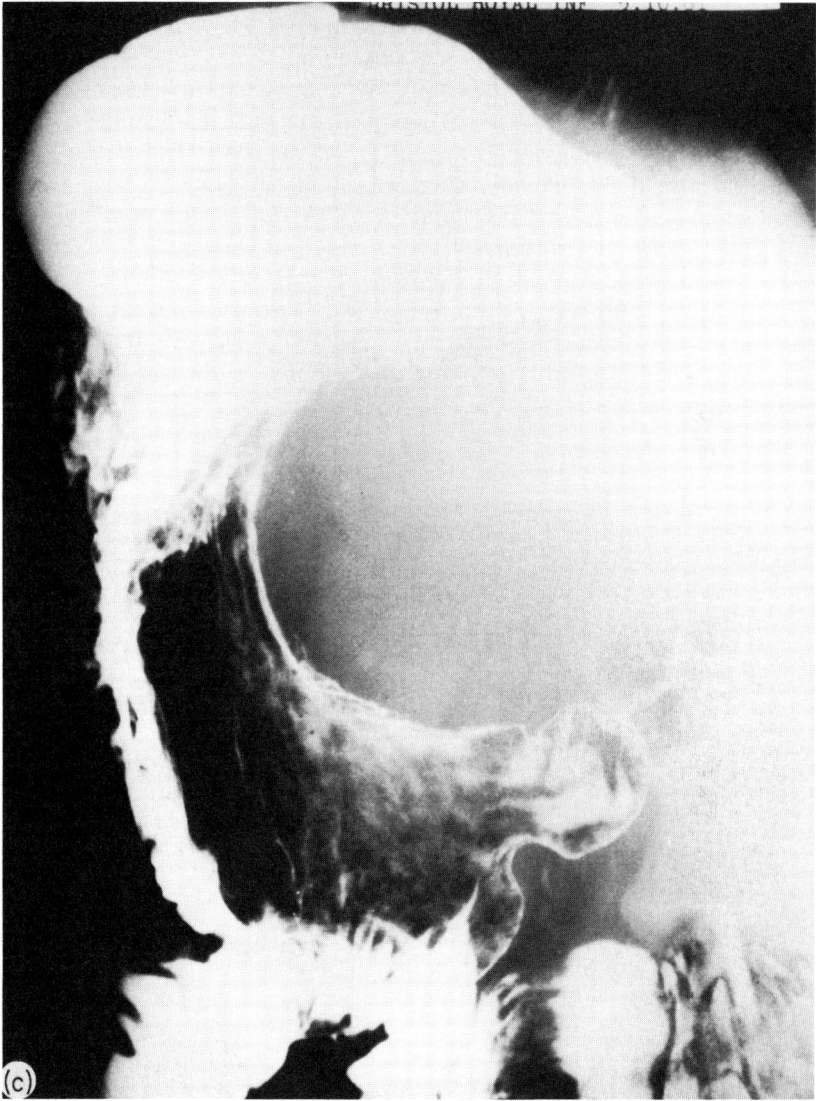

Figure 9. (a) Ultrasound scan showing a pancreatic pseudocyst in a 25-year-old man two weeks after an attack of acute alcoholic pancreatitis. (b) CT scan in the same patient showing the pseudocyst adjacent to the head and neck of pancreas. (c) Barium meal radiograph in the same patient. Oblique films show anterior displacement of the stomach by a retrogastric mass.

1984). I doubt whether these procedures are superior to operation. I would prefer to wait for 4–6 weeks and then perform internal drainage, anastomosing the mature cyst wall to a Roux loop of jejunum; the cyst is entered through the transverse mesocolon. To my mind, cystgastrostomy is less satisfactory; the cyst may not be closely applied to the back of the stomach or may extend for some distance below its lower border, and complications such as bleeding and gastric fistula may be more common (Frey, 1978; Schattenkerk et al, 1982).

Whereas pseudocysts can be left to ripen, the development of pancreatic abscess is an indication for prompt and radical surgery (Becker et al, 1984). The diagnosis is suggested by hectic fever, rising leucocytosis and deteriorating health; it is best confirmed by CT scan (Figure 10). At laparotomy the retroperitoneum must be opened widely, with removal of necrotic fat and exploration of the pancreatic bed by an infracolic approach (Shi et al, 1984). The slough can extend forwards into the root of the mesentery and transverse mesolocon, upwards towards the diaphragm, laterally around the left kidney

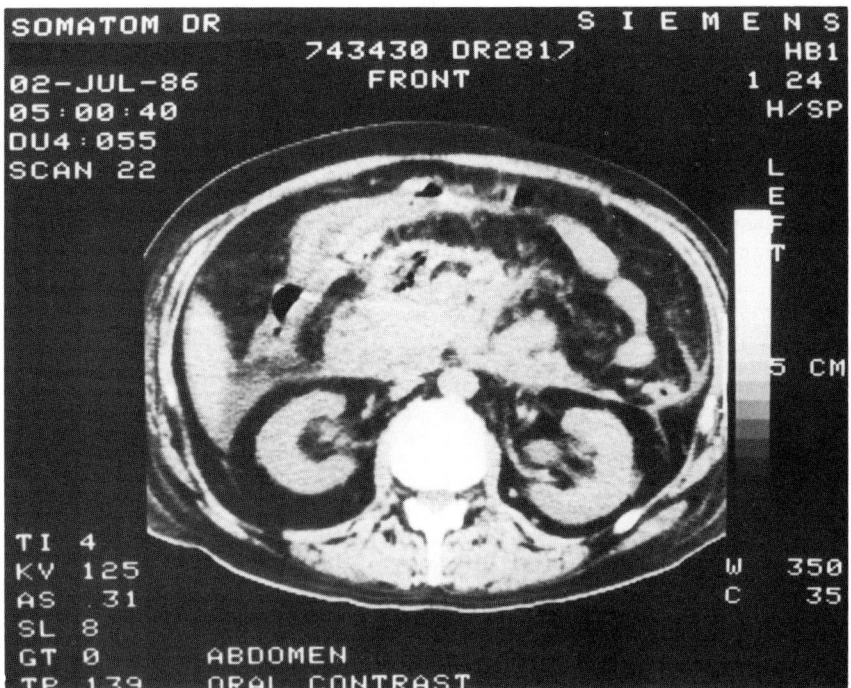

Figure 10. CT scan showing a large pancreatic abscess in a 68-year-old man three weeks after the onset of symptoms of acute pancreatitis. Following laparotomy and radical drainage he developed disseminated intravascular coagulation and eventually died despite a second drainage procedure.

and downwards behind the descending colon; debridement should be tailored accordingly (Stricker and Hunt, 1986). Haemostasis can sometimes be troublesome, and fresh frozen plasma may be needed to correct a coagulopathy. At the end of the operation several widebore drains should be placed to the abscess cavity, and it is our practice to commence postoperative lavage the following day and continue until the return fluid begins to clear. An interesting alternative is the "battlefield surgery" technique of laparotomy, in which the abdomen is left open and evisceration is prevented by the use of moist packs. Repeated exploration of the abdomen can be undertaken and any collections drained without the need for formal operation. Bradley managed 21 patients by this open method with a commendably low mortality rate (14%), though complications were numerous (Bradley and Fulenwider, 1984). A recent series of 18 laparotomies in Manchester included four patients with pancreatic abscess (Mughal et al, 1986).

Following drainage operations for pseudocyst or abscess, bleeding can occur into the gut, into the abdominal cavity or down a drainage tube. The bleeding is often profuse and can be the terminal event in a severely ill patient (Stroud et al, 1981). It usually follows erosion of a major artery, such as the splenic artery. The only alternative to laparotomy is transcatheter embolisation of the affected vessel (Huizinga et al, 1984).

Conclusion

The incidence of acute pancreatitis is increasing in Britain. The overall mortality rate stands unchanged at about 20%, reflecting the frequency with which elderly patients are affected. Hyperamylasaemia remains the diagnostic hallmark. Gallstones underlie at least half the cases, but it may require a diligent search to demonstrate their presence. In Bristol, alcoholism has become more common as a predisposing cause but still only accounts for about 10% of cases.

An early attempt should be made to separate patients with good and bad prognoses. Since clinical assessment within the first 48 hours is inadequate in this respect, objective laboratory criteria should be sought. Inspection of the peritoneal fluid obtained by paracentesis can provide a much quicker answer, but there is a small risk of visceral puncture and the technique may not be justified unless the clinician intends to act upon the findings.

Operations in acute pancreatitis can be diagnostic, prophylactic, therapeutic or in response to complications such as pseudocyst or abscess. Of these types only therapeutic operations have yet to prove their value. Urgent sphincterotomy, whether operative or endoscopic, might prevent harmful progression of the pathological changes in the pancreas. Total or subtotal pancreatectomy can salvage some dying patients, but others are killed and there is a high complication rate. In neither case it is established whether the benefits of urgent operation outweigh the substantial risks involved.

References

Acosta JM, Rossi R and Ledesma CL (1977) The usefulness of stool screening for diagnosing cholelithiasis in acute pancreatitis. A description of the technique. *Am. J. Dig. Dis.* **22**, 168–72.

Acosta JM, Rossi R, Galli OMR, Pellegrini CA and Skinner DB (1978) Early surgery for acute gallstone pancreatitis: evaluation of a systematic approach. *Surgery* **83**, 367–70.

Armstrong CP, Taylor TV, Jeacock J and Lucas S (1985) The biliary tract in patients with acute gallstone pancreatitis. *Br. J. Surg.* **72**, 551–5.

Becker JM, Pemberton JH, Di Magno EP et al (1984) Prognostic factors in pancreatic abscess. *Surgery* **96**, 455–61.

Bernardino ME and Amerson JR (1984) Percutaneous gastrocystostomy: a new approach to pancreatic pseudocyst drainage. *Am. J. Roentgenol.* **143**, 1096–7.

Berry AR, Taylor TV and Davies GC (1981) Pulmonary function and fibrinogen metabolism in acute pancreatitis. *Br. J. Surg.* **68**, 870–3.

Berry AR, Taylor TV and Davies GC (1982) Diagnostic tests and prognostic indicators in acute pancreatitis. *J. Roy. Coll. Surg. Edin.* **27**, 345–52.

Blamey SL, Imrie CW, O'Neill J, Gilmour WH and Carter DC (1984) Prognostic factors in acute pancreatitis. *Gut* **25**, 1340–6.

Bouchier IAD (1985) Biochemical tests for acute pancreatitis. *Br. Med. J.* **291**, 1669–70.

Bourke JB, Giggs JA and Ebdon DS (1979) Variations in the incidence and the spatial distribution of patients with primary acute pancreatitis in Nottingham 1969–76. *Gut* **20**, 366–71.

Bradley EL and Fulenwider JT (1984) Open treatment of pancreatic abscess. *Surg. Gynecol. Obstet.* **159**, 509–13.

Colhoun E, Murphy JJ and MacErlean DP (1984) Percutaneous drainage of pancreatic pseudocysts. *Br. J. Surg.* **71**, 131–2.

Cooper MJ, Williamson RCN and Pollock AV (1982) The role of peritoneal lavage in the prediction and treatment of severe acute pancreatitis. *Ann. Roy. Coll. Surg. Engl.* **64**, 422–7.

Corfield AP, Cooper MJ and Williamson RCN (1985a) Acute pancreatitis: a lethal disease of increasing incidence. *Gut* **26**, 724–9.

Corfield AP, Cooper MJ, Williamson RCN et al (1985b) Prediction of severity in acute pancreatitis: prospective comparison of three prognostic indices. *Lancet* **ii**, 403–7.

Cotton PB (1980) Congenital anomaly of pancreas divisum as cause of obstructive pain and pancreatitis. *Gut* **21**, 104–14.

Dammann HG, Grabbe E and Runge M (1980) Computed tomography and acute pancreatitis *Lancet* **ii**, 860.

De Bolla AR and Obeid ML (1984) Mortality in acute pancreatitis. *Ann. Roy. Coll. Surg. Engl.* **66**, 184–6.

Feller ER (1984) Endoscopic retrograde cholangiopancreatography in the diagnosis of unexplained pancreatitis. *Arch. Intern. Med.* **144**, 1797–9.

Frey CF (1978) Pancreatic pseudocyst—operative strategy. *Ann. Surg.* **188**, 652–2.

Gillat DA, Cooper MJ and Williamson RCN (1986) Pseudo-pseudocysts of the pancreas. *Pancreas* **1**, 460–3.

Hill MC, Barkin J, Isikoff MB, Silverstein W and Kalser M (1982) Acute pancreatitis: clinical vs. CT findings. *Am. J. Roentgenol.* **139**, 263–9.

Huizinga WKJ, Kalideen JM, Bryer JV, Bell PSH and Baker LW (1984) Control of major haemorrhage associated with pancreatic pseudocysts by transcatheter arterial embolization. *Br. J. Surg.* **71**, 133–6.

Ihse I, Evander A, Holmberg JT and Gustafson I (1986) Influence of peritoneal lavage on objective prognostic signs in acute pancreatitis. *Ann. Surg.* **204**, 122–7.

Imrie CW and Shearer MG (1986) Diagnosis and management of severe acute pancreatitis. In Russell RCG (ed.) *Recent Advances in Surgery 12* pp 143–154, Edinburgh: Churchill Livingstone.

Imrie CW, Benjamin IS, Ferguson JC et al. (1978a) A single-centre double-blind trial of Trasylol therapy in primary acute pancreatitis. *Br. J. Surg.* **65**, 337–41.

Imrie CW, McKay AJ, Benjamin IS and Blumgart LH (1978b) Secondary acute pancreatitis: aetiology, prevention, diagnosis and management. *Br. J. Surg.* **65**, 399–402.

Jacobs ML, Daggett WM, Civetta JM et al (1977) Acute pancreatitis: analysis of factors influencing survival. *Ann. Surg.* **185**, 43–51.

James O, Agnew JE and Bouchier IAD (1974) Chronic pancreatitis in England: a changing picture? *Br. Med. J.* **2**, 34–8.

Kelly TR (1980) Gallstone pancreatitis: the timing of surgery. *Surgery* **88**, 345–50.

Kelly TR (1984) Gallstone pancreatitis: local predisposing factors. *Ann. Surg.* **200**, 479–85.

Kivilaasko E, Fraki O and Nikki P (1981) Resection of the pancreas for acute fulminant pancreatitis. *Surg. Gynecol. Obstet.* **152**, 493–8.

Kozarek RA, Brayko CM, Harlan J et al (1985) Endoscopic drainage of pancreatic pseudocysts. *Gastrointest. Endosc.* **31**, 322–8.

Lawson DW, Daggett WM, Civetta JM, Corry RJ and Bartlett MK (1970) Surgical treatment of acute necrotizing pancreatitis. *Ann. Surg.* **172**, 605–17.

Mayer AD, McMahon MJ, Benson EA and Axon ATR (1984) Operations upon the biliary tract in patients with acute pancreatitis: aims, indications and timing. *Ann. Roy. Coll. Surg. Engl.* **66**, 179–83.

Mayer AD, McMahon MJ, Corfield AP et al (1985) Controlled clinical trial of peritoneal lavage for the treatment of severe acute pancreatitis. *New Engl. J. Med.* **312**, 399–404.

McMahon MJ (1986) Acute pancreatitis. *Current Opinion in Gastroenterology* **2**, 695–710.

McMahon MJ, Playforth MJ and Pickford IR (1980) A comparative study of methods for the prediction of severity of attacks of acute pancreatitis. *Br. J. Surg.* **67**, 22–5.

MRC Multicentre Trial (1977) Death from acute pancreatitis. *Lancet* **ii**, 632–5.

Mughal MM, Bancewicz J and Irving MH (1986) Laparostomy: a technique for the management of intractable intra-abdominal sepsis. *Br. J. Surg.* **73**, 253–9.

Nordback IH and Auvinen OA (1985) Long-term results after pancreas resection for acute necrotizing pancreatitis. *Br. J. Surg.* **72**, 687–9.

Nordback IH, Pessi T, Auvinen OA and Autio V (1985) Determination of necrosis in necrotizing pancreatitis. *Br. J. Surg.* **72**, 225–7.

Norton L and Eiseman B (1974) Near total pancreatectomy for haemorrhagic pancreatitis. *Am. J. Surg.* **127**, 191–5.

O'Malley VP, Cannon JP and Postier RG (1985) Pancreatic pseudocysts: cause, therapy, and results. *Am. J. Surg.* **150**, 680–2.

Opie EL (1901) The etiology of acute hemorrhagic pancreatitis. *Bull Johns Hopkins Hosp.* **12**, 182–8.

Osborne DH, Imrie CW and Carter DC (1981) Biliary surgery in the same admission for gallstone-associated acute pancreatitis. *Br. J. Surg.* **68**, 758–61.

Pickford IR, Blackett RJ and McMahon MJ (1977) Early assessment of severity of acute pancreatitis using peritoneal lavage. *Br. Med. J.* **2**, 1377–9.

Ranson JHC (1979) The timing of biliary surgery in acute pancreatitis. *Ann. Surg.* **189**, 654–63.

Ranson JHC and Spencer FC (1978) The role of peritoneal lavage in severe acute pancreatitis. *Ann. Surg.* **187**, 565–75.

Ranson JHC, Rifkind KM, Roses DF et al (1974) Prognostic signs and the role of operative management in acute pancreatitis. *Surg. Gynecol. Obstet.* **139**, 69–81.

Ranson JHC, Rifkind KM and Turner JW (1976) Prognostic signs and nonoperative peritoneal lavage in acute pancreatitis. *Surg. Gynec. Obstet.* **143**, 209–19.

Renner IG, Savage WT III, Pantoja JL and Renner VJ (1985) Death due to acute pancreatitis. A retrospective analysis of 405 autopsy cases. *Dig. Dis. Sci.* **30**, 1005–18.

Rose DM, Ranson JHC, Cunningham JN Jr and Spencer FC (1984) Patterns of severe pancreatic injury following cardiopulmonary bypass. *Ann. Surg.* **199**, 168–72.

Rosseland AR and Solhaug JH (1984) Early or delayed endoscopic papillotomy (EPT) in gallstone pancreatitis. *Ann. Surg.* **199**, 165–7.

Safrany L and Cotton PB (1981) A preliminary report: urgent duodenoscopic sphincterotomy for acute gallstone pancreatitis. *Surgery* **89**, 424–8.

Satiani S and Stone HH (1979) Predictability of present outcome and future recurrence in acute pancreatitis. *Arch. Surg.* **114**, 711–6.

Schattenkerk M E, De Vries JE, Bruining HA, Eggink WF and Obertop H (1982) Surgical treatment of pancreatic pseudocysts. *Br. J. Surg.* **69**, 593–4.

Schein M, Saadia R and Decker G (1985) Colonic necrosis in acute pancreatitis. A complication of massive retroperitoneal suppuration. *Dis. Colon Rectum* **28**, 948–50.

Shi ECP, Yeo BW and Ham JM (1984) Pancreatic abscesses. *Br. J. Surg.* **71**, 689–91.

Smadja C and Bismuth H (1984) Acute necrotising pancreatitis: towards restriction in surgery. *Gastroenterol. Clin. Biol.* **8**, 536–40.

Spuy S van der (1981) Endoscopic sphincterotomy in the management of gallstone pancreatitis. *Endoscopy* **13**, 25–6.

Stone HH and Fabian TC (1980) Peritoneal dialysis in the treatment of acute alcoholic pancreatitis. *Surg. Gynec. Obstet.* **150**, 878–82.

Stone HH, Fabian TC and Dunlop WE (1981) Gallstone pancreatitis. Biliary tract pathology in relation to time of operation. *Ann. Surg.* **194**, 305–12.

Stone HH, Mullins RJ and Scovill WA (1985) Vagotomy plus Billroth II gastrectomy for the prevention of recurrent alcohol-induced pancreatitis. *Ann. Surg.* **201**, 684–9.

Stricker PD and Hunt DR (1986) Surgical aspects of pancreatic abscess. *Br. J. Surg.* **73**, 644–6.

Stroud WH, Cullom JW and Anderson MC (1981) Hemorrhagic complications of severe pancreatitis. *Surgery* **90**, 657–65.

Trapnell JE (1966) Natural history and prognosis of acute pancreatitis. *Am. Roy. Coll. Surg. Engl.* **38**, 265–87.

Trapnell JE and Duncan EHL (1975) Patterns of incidence in acute pancreatitis. *Br. Med. J.* **2**, 179–83.

Warshaw AL and Jin G (1985) Improved survival in 45 patients with pancreatic abscess. *Ann. Surg.* **202,** 408–17.

Watts GT (1963) Total pancreatectomy for fulminant pancreatitis. *Lancet* **ii**, 384.

Williamson RCN (1984) Early assessment of severity in acute pancreatitis. *Gut* **25**, 1331–9.

Key Developments in Gastroenterology
Edited by P. R. Salmon
© 1988 John Wiley & Sons Ltd

9

Campylobacter: Is it Important?

D. G. Colin-Jones

Queen Alexandra Hospital, Portsmouth, Hampshire

Could peptic ulcers be caused by an infection? Should we now equate all that data on acid with earlier views on stress, and relegate it to the category, 'interesting, but passé? The recently identified organism, *Campylobacter pylori* (CP), has generated much interest and raised many questions. It is remarkable for its high degree of adaptation as it seems to be found exclusively on human gastric mucosa on the surface of the epithelial cells and deep to the mucus. It has been found in a high proportion of cases both with gastritis and with peptic ulcer—which has raised considerable speculation as to whether peptic ulceration is in reality an infection (Axon, 1986). Will peptic ulcer treatment of tomorrow be an antibiotic?

Historical Aspects

The organism, currently called *Campylobacter pylori* (CP), is probably a new genus, although it was first observed as long ago as 1906. It was documented in the human stomach in 1940 by Freedberg and Barron. My first link with this organism was in 1975 when working with Howard Steer (Steer and Colin-Jones, 1975). We wondered whether bacteria might contribute to ulcers by damaging mucus and so predisposing to penetration of acid and, from that, ulceration. We therefore took multiple biopsies from a large number of gastric ulcer patients and found these curious Gram-negative bacteria deep to the mucus and on the surface of the epithelium (Figure 1), which in retrospect were undoubtedly CP. At that time culture media were not readily available because this organism is slow-growing and rather fastidious. It was in 1984 that Marshall and Warren (Marshall and Warren, 1984) successfully cultured and then described these S-shaped, spiral bacteria which are Gram-negative and appear to have 4–6 sheathed flagella, each with a small terminal bulb—unlike other Campylobacters. Although it has some of the features of the genus *Campylobacter*, CP is not nitrate-reducing and has a remarkable capacity for

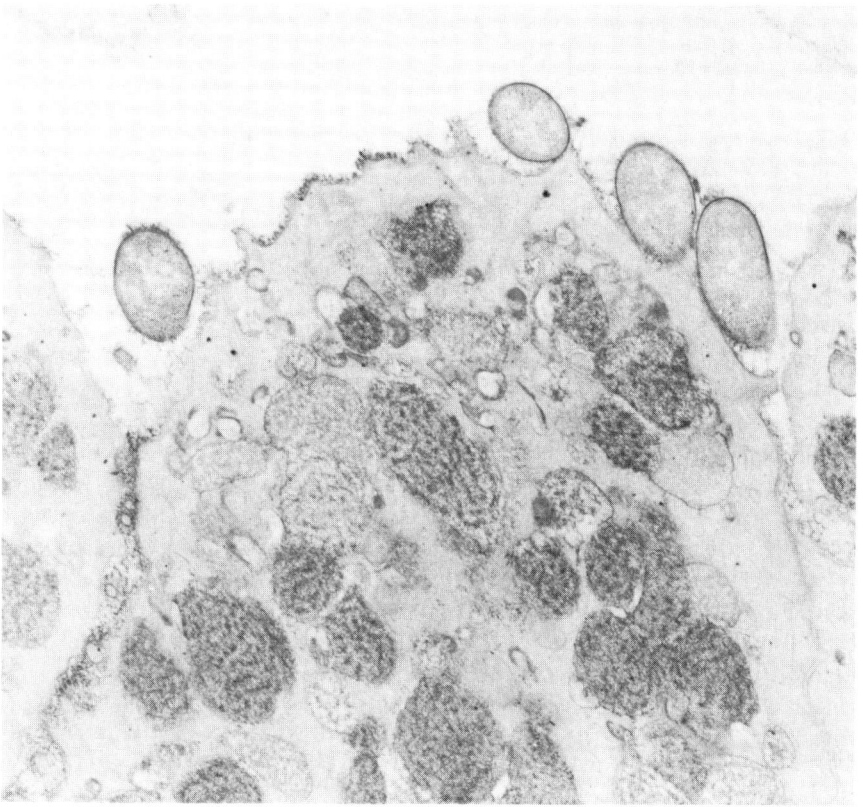

Figure 1. Electron micrograph of the surface of the gastric mucosa, showing CP adherent to the cell wall and tending to enter the gutters between the mucosal cells.

splitting urea—features not found in other Campylobacters. The capacity for splitting urea is so marked that a homogenised biopsy, with measurement of urease activity, can be used to determine whether or not the sample contains CP. The majority of the cellular fatty acids also are different from those of most pathogenic Campylobacter species. The organism is slow to grow in culture. It is not found in gastric aspirate because it lives deep to the mucus layer. However, gastric biopsies can be cultured in media suitable for other Campylobacters, or it may be identified by means of electron microscopy or special stains, such as the Warthin-Starry silver stain. The simplest technique is a modified Giemsa which is substantially easier and cheaper than the Warthin-Starry. In the future it may be possible to identify the presence of the organism by the presence of circulating antibodies (Rathbone et al, 1986).

Gastritis

Gastritis has several causes. The so-called type A is autoimmune gastritis associated with pernicious anaemia. Much more commonly there is type B gastritis which is non-immune. This may be caused by a number of factors such as bile reflux. The non-autoimmune type of gastritis is strongly associated with the presence of CP, which usually colonises the gastric antrum in non-acid-secreting mucosa and may also be found in more proximal gastric biopsies where there is a gastritis. However, areas of intestinal metaplasia are not colonised, and perhaps even more remarkably ectopic gastric epithelium in the duodenal cap is colonised by CP, whereas the more normal intestinal type of duodenal mucosa is not affected. The organisms are located particularly in the gutters between epithelial cells where they adhere to the cell surface and cause a pseudopodium-like structure (Figure 1) to which they are adherent. An acute inflammatory reaction follows the presence of this organism and there is a high correlation between inflammatory infiltrate and CP infection. As one might expect, antibodies are raised by the host to the organism, although some individuals appear to be unable to eradicate the organism from the stomach. The antibodies are specific and found in the IgG and IgA class, and using immunoperoxidase techniques antibodies have been shown to coat the organisms, although not those very deep in the gutters between cells (a location they seem to prefer) (Figure 2), where they seem to be protected from antibody.

Acute gastritis

Several reports in the literature point to an epidemic achlorhydria, with an associated acute gastritis. This has been documented by two research groups in which volunteers appear to have been contaminated by an infecting agent transmitted through an electrode, with consequent reduction in gastric acid secretion, an acute gastritis and symptoms of nausea and anorexia. In the majority of volunteers the effects gradually cleared but in some they persisted for several months. CP could fit well with such an infecting agent. Support for this comes from a study in which Marshall took 10^9 organisms, having demonstrated that his stomach was normal by endoscopy and biopsy and had not previously been colonised by CP (Marshall et al, 1985a). Following ingestion of these organisms he felt generally nauseated, with borborygmi, abdominal discomfort, distension and halitosis. On day 10 these spiral organisms were present. There was a reduction in the intracellular mucus and a heavy infiltrate of polymorphs in the mucosa. On electron microscopy the microvilli were depleted. Four days later he had already begun to feel better and the biopsy showed no evidence of any organisms and the polymorphonuclear infiltrate had diminished. Although the mucus content of the cells had improved this was an incomplete recovery. Marshall then took an antibiotic but in fact eradication of the organisms had

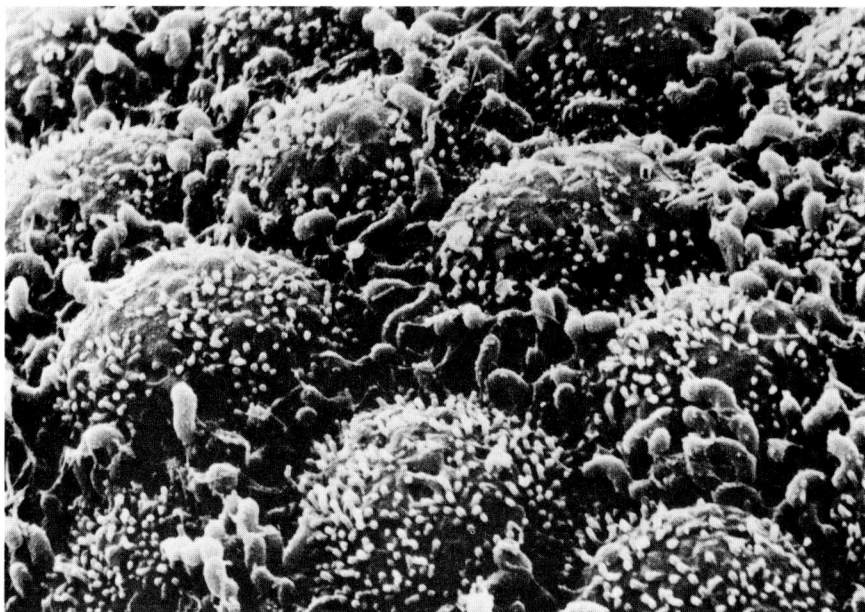

Figure 2 Scanning electron micrograph in a patient with a duodenal ulcer, showing numerous organisms colonising the surface especially in the gutters between cells. Reproduced by permission of H.W. Steer and the Editor of *Gut*.

already occurred prior to its ingestion. CP undoubtedly causes an acute gastritis, and may well persist to cause a chronic gastritis in susceptible people.

Chronic gastritis

Normal people

Normal volunteers with absolutely no gastric symptoms have had gastroscopies. In one group, 6 out of 25 healthy medical students were found to have a chronic gastritis with the organism present but they had no symptoms. The organism is seldom found except when gastritis is present. This absence of symptoms is a complicating factor in our understanding of the relationship between CP and dyspepsia.

Dyspeptic patients

In an important study by McNulty and colleagues (1986) dyspeptic patients who were undergoing gastroscopy as part of their investigation were studied for the presence of this organism. Those who had dyspepsia and CP present (but no ulcer) were treated either with bismuth, erythromycin or a placebo, the organism having previously been found to be sensitive to both bismuth and a number of antibiotics, including erythromycin. Interestingly, 14 of 18 patients receiving bismuth salicylate cleared the organism but only 1 of 15 receiving erythromycin, and none of 18 patients taking placebo. CP was cleared, then, in 15 patients, of whom 13 had gastritis and this resolved in 12. Conversely, the gastritis resolved in only 4 of 32 patients in whom the organism was not eradicated. Of 12 patients with symptoms whose organism was cleared, 11 noted a symptomatic improvement, which compared with 21 improved out of 32 (66%) in those with persistent infection. Thus although removal of the organism results in a considerable improvement in the histological appearances and some benefits symptomatically, not all patients obtain symptom relief. Sadly, recolonisation by this organism seems to be common.

Bile reflux gastritis

The other major cause of non-autoimmune gastritis is enterogastric reflux. This particularly occurs after gastric surgery and increases in severity and extent with time after the operation. Where enterogastric reflux occurs infrequently, such as in the unoperated stomach of a duodenal patient or after a highly selective vagotomy, one would expect a high incidence of CP and this was indeed found (97% and 94%) by O'Connor et al (1986). However, the frequency with which the organism was found following operations in which bile reflux was common, was much lower—22% after a Billroth I gastrectomy, 47% after a Billroth II gastrectomy and 50% after a truncal vagotomy and gastroenterostomy. There was a highly significant reduction in CP positive biopsies when there was a high degree of reflux. These workers suggest that the reflux of bile may disrupt the mucus and so cause the death of any Campylobacters living beneath it but at the same time, of course, produce an inflammatory response.

Peptic ulcer

Campylobacter pylori is found in the gastric antrum of more than 90% of patients with duodenal ulcer and approximately 70% to 80% of patients with gastric ulcer. It has been suggested that the organism contributes to the development of an ulcer by its urease activity producing large quantities of ammonia deep to the mucus layer which, by altering the pH, changes the permeability of the mucosa and predisposes to ulceration (Hazell and Lee, 1986).

The first clue that this organism might be important in peptic ulceration was observed before CP was identified, as a study by Martin et al (1981), subsequently confirmed by other workers, showed that healing a duodenal ulcer with colloidal bismuth (De-Nol) led to a smaller relapse rate in subsequent months than when the original ulcer was healed with an H_2-receptor antagonist such as cimetidine or ranitidine. The finding that this organism is sensitive to bismuth—and at present this seems to be the agent of choice in eradicating the organism from the mucosa—would suggest that perhaps its eradication may reduce the relapse rate. This is supported by preliminary data presented at the World Congress of Gastroenterology at Sao Paulo, September 1986, by Marshall, who reported a trial in which he treated a group of duodenal ulcer patients for 56 days with a combination of bismuth and tinidazole (an antibiotic to which CP is sensitive in vitro) or placebo. Forty-three patients healed their ulcers (87% had eradicated the organism), whilst of 17 patients who did not heal their ulcers, 16 still had CP. He then followed these patients for 6 months; 21 became reinfected with a 92% recurrence of ulcer, 12 remained free of CP on biopsy and they had only a 27% recurrence. These are important data which need confirmation in larger studies but suggest that CP plays a role in ulcer disease.

The mechanism by which CP might contribute to ulceration involves several possibilities. In the initial infection hypochlorhydria may well be produced but this gradually reverses. But as acid secretion recovers, the mucosa, especially in the antrum and where there is ectopic gastric epithelium in the duodenal cap, is now chronically inflamed with an inflammatory cell infiltrate. The surface cells are disorganised—the mucosal barrier, so-called, has been disrupted. Furthermore the mucus blanket covering the epithelium, which maintains a pH gradient at the epithelial cell surface, may well be diminished in patients colonised by this organism, as it produces a disturbance of enterocyte mucus production. Then, as indicated already, the urease activity with ammonia production has been postulated as causing local damage with further impairment of the mucosal defences. Acid and pepsin are probably the final insult to the mucosa which lead to the development of the ulcer.

Other Organisms

Most attention has focused on CP but other organisms have been identified in almost identical locations—deep to the mucus and in the gastric antrum. It may well be that, although the majority of cases involve CP, some patients have similar but different organisms producing pathology.

Discussion

It is less than four years since CP was first identified and the interest it has aroused has been tremendous, with many groups looking at a wide variety of aspects, trying to establish whether or not this organism is clinically important. The evidence that CP causes a high proportion of non-autoimmune gastritis is overwhelming. The problem, however, is that whilst in some cases this seems to produce symptoms, in others it does not and the host is quite unaware that he or she has such an infection. When it comes to studying the relationship between CP and ulcers, there again is a high correlation between the presence of an ulcer and the presence of this organism but the correlation does not necessarily mean that CP causes ulcers.

Koch proposed four postulates which, if confirmed, would prove that a particular organism was responsible for a particular disease. His first postulate was that the organisms should always be found microscopically in the bodies of animals having the disease and in that disease only. It should occur in such numbers and be distributed in such a manner as to explain the lesions of that disease. As indicated by Marshall et al (1985a), the non-autoimmune gastritis fulfils this postulate. It seems probable that the majority (but not all) of cases of type B gastritis are associated with CP. However, this is not the case for peptic ulcer disease. CP is found predominantly in the gastric antrum and on islands of ectopic gastric epithelium in the duodenal cap, but the ulcer is located away from the main area of infection.

The second postulate was that the organism should be obtained from the diseased animal and grown outside the body. This criterion has been satisfied especially for gastritis but also in the majority of cases of duodenal ulcer. The frequency with which CP is demonstrated in proximity to gastric ulcers is somewhat lower, but still high at 70–80%.

The third postulate proposed by Koch was that the inoculation of these germs in pure culture, freed by successive transplantations from the smallest particle of matter taken from the original animal, should produce the same disease in a susceptible animal. As indicated above, this organism was inoculated into a volunteer—Dr Marshall himself—and this produced an acute gastritis. It is yet to be demonstrated that this will proceed to a chronic gastritis or indeed to an ulcer. The third postulate has therefore not been fulfilled for chronic gastritis or ulcer disease.

The fourth postulate is that the germ should be found in the diseased areas so produced in the animal. This criterion has been fulfilled by Dr Marshall's experiment as his stomach was colonised by CP. The same experiment has not been done in peptic ulcer disease.

It is clear that Koch's postulates for the association between CP and gastritis have very nearly been fulfilled, whilst those for peptic ulcer are still a long way from proof. However, the theoretical basis by which CP causes gastric damage makes it very attractive as a factor in ulcer disease. It causes an inflammatory reaction, disorganisation of the cellular structure on the surface of the epithelium, and then reduces the mucus production which could well allow acid present to penetrate more readily. There are, however, many unknowns. If CP is important in ulcer disease, why is it located primarily in the gastric antrum and less heavily in the duodenum which is the commonest site of ulceration? For gastritis there is the problem of correlation with symptoms which is poor.

In the past we have probably been too simplistic in our approach to ulcer disease because acid and pepsin seem to be involved and probably complete the disease process, since the dictum 'no acid, no ulcer' still applies. However, peptic ulcers probably have several different causes. In some there is good evidence of hypersecretion of acid as the major factor. There is considerable interest at the moment in pepsin, with an increase in pepsin 2 being found in some duodenal ulcer sufferers. Other patients—especially the elderly—probably have the effects of non-steroidal anti-inflammatory drugs as the major contributor to their ulcers. In others there may be, for example, prostaglandin deficiency, which has been documented in some ulcers; there may be a pharmacological effect from smoking, which at the moment has not been discovered; and diet and stress may of course contribute, although this is conjectural. I would put *Campylobacter pylori* along with these many other factors as it would appear to be an important contributor to the breakdown of the mucosal defence, which then allows acid to cause the final damage, producing ulceration. Much work needs to be done to confirm this hypothesis and to determine the proportion of patients whose ulcer is initiated by this infection.

References

Axon ATR (1986) *Campylobacter pyloridis*: what role in gastritis and peptic ulcer? *Br. Med. J.* **293**, 772–3.

Hazell SL and Lee A (1986) *Campylobacter pyloridis*, urease, hydrogen ion back diffusion, and gastric ulcers. *Lancet* **ii**, 15–17.

Marshall BJ and Warren JR (1984) Unidentified curved bacilli in the stomach of patients with gastritis and peptic ulceration. *Lancet* **i**, 1311–4.

Marshall BJ, Armstrong JA, McGechie DB and Glancy RJ (1985a) Attempt to fulfil Koch's postulates for pyloric campylobacter. *Med. J. Aust.* **142**, 436–9.

Marshall BJ, McGechie DB, Rogers PA and Glancy RJ (1985b) Pyloric *Campylobacter* infection and gastroduodenal disease. *Med. J. Aust.* **142**, 439–44.

Martin DF, Hollanders D, May SJ et al (1981) Difference in relapse rates of duodenal ulcer after healing with cimetidine or tripotassium dicitrato bismuthate. *Lancet* **i**, 7–10.

McNulty C, Gearty JC, Crump B et al (1986) *Campylobacter pyloridis* and associated gastritis: investigator blind, placebo controlled trial of bismuth salicylate and erythromycin ethylsuccinate. *Br. Med. J.* **293**, 645–9.

O'Connor HJ, Dixon MF, Wyatt JI et al (1986) Effect of duodenal ulcer surgery and enterogastric reflux on *Campylobacter pyloridis. Lancet* **ii**, 1178–81.

Rathbone BJ, Wyatt JI and Heatley RV (1986) *Campylobacter pyloridis*—a new factor in peptic ulcer disease? *Gut* **27**, 635–41.

Steer HW (1984) Surface morphology of the gastroduodenal mucosa in duodenal ulceration. *Gut* **25**, 1203–10.

Steer HW and Colin-Jones DG (1975) Mucosal changes in gastric ulceration and their response to carbenoxolone sodium. *Gut* **16**, 590–7.

Key Developments in Gastroenterology
Edited by P. R. Salmon
© 1988 John Wiley & Sons Ltd

10

Non-steroidal Drug-induced Gastric Damage

M. J. S. Langman

Queen Elizabeth Hospital, Birmingham

There has been widespread clinical suspicion that non-aspirin non-steroidal anti-inflammatory drugs (NANSAIDs) cause peptic ulceration, and that they do so commonly and to a clinically significant degree.

Experimental Data

Animal evidence indicates that damage, with multiple erosions occurring in the stomach, is common though generally this is less pronounced than when aspirin is employed as the damaging agent (Vakil et al, 1977; Pitts and Proctor, 1978). Effects tend to be dose-related and have been observed for all NANSAIDs. When anti-inflammatory potency is taken into account, then no fundamental differences seem to exist between individual drugs.

Experiments conducted in man likewise show that exposure to NANSAIDs is associated with gastroscopic evidence of submucosal haemorrhage and the development of mucosal erosions, a tendency for back diffusion of hydrogen ions, and microbleeding into the gastric lumen. Persuasive though this evidence may be, it does not allow direct extrapolation to ordinary peptic ulceration.

Case Series

Exposure to NANSAIDs has been associated with the occurrence of gastric ulcer (Emmanuel and Montgomery, 1971), with perforation of duodenal ulcer for indomethacin alone (Thompson, 1980) and for NANSAIDs in general (Collier and Pain, 1985), with bleeding from gastric and duodenal ulcers (O'Brien and Burnham, 1985), and in the elderly with the occurrence of both gastric and duodenal ulcers (Clinch et al, 1983). In addition, Caruso and Porro (1980) have shown a high frequency of apparently new gastroduodenal lesions in patients treated with a wide variety of NANSAIDs who were endoscoped before and after treatment. Patients exposed have generally been elderly so that, despite the high frequency with which antecedent NANSAID drug use was detected, it was impossible to say with complete confidence that treatment was causal, and the lack of control data prevented any calculations of risk. Nevertheless, patients with bleeding and perforated ulcers seemed to have levels of preceding NANSAID exposure that were distinctly higher than would have been expected from local prevailing drug prescription rates.

Case-control data

Ulcer disease in general

Clinch and his colleagues (1983) compared the frequency of antecedent NANSAID use in elderly dyspeptic individuals submitted to endoscopy and in whom peptic ulcers were and were not found. NANSAID use was much more common in those found to have gastric and duodenal ulcers. It is difficult to know what referral biases may have prevailed but the data nevertheless appeared to indicate a clinically important association. In Australia Duggan and his colleagues (1986) have compared the frequency of previous NANSAID use in patients diagnosed as having gastric or duodenal ulcers with the frequency in community controls interviewed by telephone. An increased risk of associated gastric but not duodenal ulcer was detected, although case numbers were rather small and confidence limits around estimates must inevitably be wide.

Ulcer complications

In Nottingham we compared the frequency of previous NANSAID use in patients aged 60 and over admitted with bleeding gastric and duodenal ulcers with the frequency in hospital inpatient controls admitted as medical emergencies and in community controls chosen randomly from the practice lists of the doctors responsible for the ordinary care of the patients admitted with ulcer bleeding (all United Kingdom people being registered for care with a general medical practitioner) (Somerville et al, 1986).

Patients admitted with bleeding ulcers were between two and six times as likely to be taking NANSAIDs as hospital or community controls (Table 1). Usage was markedly greater than in younger patients with bleeding and did not differ materially in those admitted with gastric ulcer and duodenal ulcer bleeding. The data obtained also suggested that the risk did not lie with individuals with destructive inflammatory arthropathies such as rheumatoid arthritis and that it was at least as obvious in association with short-term treatment as long-term treatment. Data obtained, if assumed to be generalisable to the United Kingdom overall, were compatible with the suggestion that some 2000 admissions with bleeding were caused by treatment with NANSAIDs and at least 200 deaths assuming, at a conservative estimate, a 10% death rate.

Table 1. Outcome of questioning about NANSAID intake by patients with upper gastrointestinal bleeding and by controls (Somerville et al, 1986).

Patients	Controls	
with bleeding	Hospital inpatient	Community
80	33	34
150	197	173
230	227	207
% users:		
Relative risk (compared with controls)	3.8	2.7
95% confidence limits	2.2–6.4	1.7–4.4

Assuming a similar risk for ulcer perforation would imply an extra 400 to 500 cases induced.

Surveillance data

Two large surveillance series have been reported. In the first (Inman, 1984), outcome was studied in five groups of approximately 10 000 individuals who received five different NANSAIDs (benoxaprofen, Osmosin brand indomethacin, fenbufen, zomepirac and piroxicam). By comparison with ulcer complication rates in periods without use of the drug under consideration no risk of ulcer complications was detected. In the second series conducted in California (Jick et al, 1985) a period of 90 days at risk was defined following prescription of NANSAIDs. Again, no material risk was detected for gastric ulcer in a population of all ages under 65 years.

Spontaneous adverse reaction reports

Reports on yellow cards to the United Kingdom Committee on Safety of Medicines more commonly concern NANSAIDs than any other variety of drug (CSM Update, 1986). The total number of reports of serious gastrointestinal damage each year, less than 250, is nevertheless very small in relation to the total number of NANSAID prescriptions which now amount to some 24 million each year in England and Wales. It is likely that less than 10% of all suspected drug reactions are reported. Despite the uncertainties of the data, which include biases towards the selective reporting of reactions for new rather than for old drugs, it is likely that spontaneous reports do indicate an important series of adverse reactions.

Reconciling the various sets of evidence

Whilst gastroenterologists perceive that adverse reactions to NANSAIDs are common and important, those responsible for surveillance studies see little in the way of problems, and general practitioners would comment generally on the frequency of dyspepsia, but not of ulcer complications. Data can be reconciled if the sources and the probable numbers of prescriptions leading to suspected adverse reactions are taken into account. Data obtained in Nottingham indicate that in the elderly about one-third of episodes of upper gastrointestinal bleeding from gastric or duodenal ulcer were associated with NANSAID use, or about 50 in a single year. In addition, 10% of episodes in younger patients were associated, or about 10 episodes. The total of 60 occurred in a population of about 800 000. In the UK as a whole about 24 million prescriptions are issued each year, or about 400 000 per million population, or about 600 000 in two years in Nottingham, giving rise to 60 drug-associated episodes, or about 1 per 10 000 population. Risk almost certainly differs in the young and old, being materially greater in the latter, but post-marketing surveillance has covered individuals of all ages.

A surveillance study in 10 000 people of all ages would be expected to detect one associated episode whilst a general practitioner writing 1000 prescriptions a year would not expect to see an associated episode of ulcer bleeding for about ten years. By contrast, the gastroenterologist seeing all episodes of bleeding in Nottingham sees the outcome of 300 000 prescriptions a year within the city. This, given an average prescription duration of one month's treatment, would be about 25 000 patient-years of treatment.

The calculation indicates that the gastroenterologist experiences the results of an enormous amount of prescribing, and this gives rise to the judgement that treatment is unsafe through ignoring what is safely happening in the community. The general practitioner with his smaller sample drawn from an average run of people judges the matter differently. The differing perceptions are easily understandable. Given the very large number of prescriptions the attributable risk of disease (the proportion caused by treatment) is high even though the

Table 2. Percentage change in admission rates with gastric and duodenal ulcer in England and Wales (Walt et al, 1986) between 1958–62 and 1979–82

Men		
Age (yr)	Duodenal ulcer	Gastric ulcer
15–44	−62	−86
45–64	−50	−72
65+	−13	−51

Women		
Age (yr)	Duodenal ulcer	Gastric ulcer
15–44	−36	−25
45–64	+38	−39
65+	+145	+20

relative risk (the increased chances of an individual taken getting the disease), is rather low.

In the UK as a whole admission rates with ulcer perforation have risen in the elderly in recent years (Walt et al, 1986). However, the increase which is obvious for duodenal ulcer and in elderly women (Table 2) is only likely to be partially attributable to anti-inflammatory drug use.

References

Caruso D and Porro GB (1980) Gastroscopic evaluation of anti-inflammatory drugs. *Br. Med. J.* **1**, 75–8

Clinch D, Banerjee AK, Ostick G and Levy DW (1983) Non steroidal anti-inflammatory drugs and gastro-intestinal adverse effects. *J.R. Coll. Physicians Lond.* **17**, 288–30.

Collier D St J and Pain JA (1985) Non-steroidal anti-inflammatory drugs and peptic ulcer perforation. *Gut* **26**, 359–63.

CSM Update (1986) Non-steroidal anti-inflammatory drugs and serious gastrointestinal reactions-1. *Br. Med. J.* **292**, 614.

Duggan JM, Dobson AJ, Johnson J and Fahey P (1986) Peptic ulcer and non steroidal anti-inflammatory agents. *Gut* **27**, 929–33.

Emmanuel JH and Montgomery RD (1971) Gastric ulcer and anti-arthritic drugs. *Postgrad. Med. J.* **47**, 227–32.

Inman WHW (1984) Non-steroidal anti-inflammatory drugs. *PEM News* **2**, 4–10.

Jick H, Feld AD and Perera DR (1985) Certain non-steroidal anti-inflammatory drugs and hospitalization for upper gastrointestinal bleeding. *Pharmacotherapy* **5**, 289–94.

O'Brien JD and Burnham WR (1985) Bleeding from peptic ulcers and use of non-steroidal anti-inflammatory drugs in the Romford area. *Br. Med. J.* **291**, 1609–10.

Pitts NE and Proctor RR (1978) Summary: efficacy and safety of piroxicam. *Royal Society of Medicine International Congress and Symposium Series* No. 1. 97–108.

Somerville K, Faulkner G and Langman MJS (1986) Non-steroidal anti-inflammatory drugs and bleeding peptic ulcer. *Lancet* **i**, 462–4.

Thompson MR (1980) Indomethacin and perforated duodenal ulcer. *Br. Med. J.* **280**, 448.

Vakil BJ, Kulkarni RD, Kulkarni VN et al (1977) Estimation of gastrointestinal blood loss in volunteers treated with non steroidal anti-inflammatory agents. *Curr. Med. Res. Opin.* **5**, 32.

Walt RP, Katschinski B, Logan R, Ashely J and Langman MJS (1986) Rising frequency of ulcer perforation in elderly people in the United Kingdom. *Lancet* **i**, 489–92.

Key Developments in Gastroenterology
Edited by P. R. Salmon
© 1988 John Wiley & Sons Ltd

11

Towards Optimal Control of Intragastric Acidity

R. E. Pounder

Royal Free Hospital School of Medicine, London

The discovery of the histamine H_2-receptor antagonists introduced a completely new era in the management of peptic ulceration (Black et al, 1972): for the first time physicians had the opportunity to control gastric acid secretion. Hitherto the only form of anti-secretory drug was atropine or its derivatives; the doses were very limited because of side-effects, and so were the clinical results (Ivey, 1975).

H_2-Revolution and H_2-Evolution

The first and last human experiments with burimamide showed that the drug was a potent anti-secretory agent (Wyllie et al, 1972), and preliminary trials with metiamide showed that control of gastric acid secretion was associated with both symptomatic improvement of duodenal ulceration and duodenal ulcer healing (Pounder et al, 1975a; Multicentre Trial, 1975). Metiamide was withdrawn abruptly, because the drug caused agranulocytosis in approximately 1 in 100 patients (Duncan and Parsons, 1980).

There was then a temporary halt to the clinical application of H_2-blockers until cimetidine was available for clinical trials. During this time we considered very carefully the optimum way to use the drug. It was generally thought that the very best results would be achieved by producing a maximal decrease of acidity across the 24 hours. For this reason we devised a technique of studying large numbers of patients simultaneously, which allowed careful control of environmental conditions, whilst we measured intragastric acidity on- and off-treatment with an H_2-blocker (Pounder et al, 1975b, 1976). The results of these experiments led us to believe that the most economic decrease of 24-hour intragastric acidity would be achieved by giving cimetidine 200 mg three times a day with meals, with 400 mg at night. Even today, I still believe that this is the regimen, using cimetidine, which will produce the greatest decrease of acidity, unless far higher doses of the drug are taken four times a day.

During the early development of ranitidine, it was realised that the drug was more potent than cimetidine on a milligram-for-milligram basis. This fact, combined with a potential marketing advantage of a twice daily drug regimen, resulted in the now familiar regimen using ranitidine 150 mg twice a day—first thing in the morning and at bedtime (Walt et al, 1981). It is interesting to note that this regimen produces inhibition of secretion during the early part of the day and also during the night—but it actually has very little effect on intragastric acidity in the late afternoon and early evening.

I think it was the potential threat of omeprazole (Clissola and Campoli-Richards, 1986), a drug that can be taken once a day, together with the knowledge that once-a-day maintenance treatment actually keeps most ulcer patients in remission (Burland et al, 1980), that provoked the next step. This was to test single doses of H_2-blockers at bedtime, in terms of 24-hour acidity profiles (Gledhill et al, 1983), and also to test such drug regimens by therapeutic trial (Ireland et al, 1984; Ryan et al, 1986; Delattre et al, 1985; Capurso et al, 1984; Lee et al, 1986). Either ranitidine 300 mg at bedtime or cimetidine 800 mg at bedtime causes a very profound decrease of nocturnal intragastric acidity which continues to the following morning (Gledhill et al, 1983). On both of these regimens intragastric acidity is essentially unchanged for most of the daytime and early evening, yet clinical trials show that this pulse of inhibition does produce duodenal ulcer healing, very similar to the traditional multiple dose regimens that had been used hitherto (Ireland et al, 1984; Ryan et al, 1986; Delattre et al, 1985; Capurso et al, 1984; Lee et al, 1986). It is hoped that a once-daily regimen improves compliance, and this improvement is probably balanced by a potential decrease of effectiveness due to lack of control of acidity during the day.

Others might also argue that the night is the most important part of the 24 hours—Professor Hunt and his colleagues from Canada have assimilated the data of many 24-hour experiments, comparing this data with the results of clinical trials, and have shown that there is a strong positive correlation between the degree of inhibition of nocturnal acidity by an H_2-blocker and the four-week ulcer healing rate (Hunt et al, 1986). However, it must be noted, when looking at these data, that extension of the regression lines so that H_2-blockers cause a 100% decrease of nocturnal acidity produces an ulcer healing rate of approximately 80% per month—that is, if one controls only nocturnal acidity, albeit infinitely, one can still only heal four out of five ulcers!

Omeprazole, the hydrogen potassium ATPase inhibitor (Clissola et al, 1986), when given in a dose of 20–30 mg each morning, produces a virtual 100% inhibition of 24-hour intragastric acidity (Sharma et al, 1984a; Pritchard et al, 1983; Lanzon-Miller et al, 1987a), and it also achieves virtual 100% ulcer healing after four weeks of treatment (Cooperative Study, 1984; Gustavsson et al, 1983; Bardram et al, 1986; Lauritsen et al, 1985). Thus it does seem that eliminating acidity, both by day and by night, is able to improve the ulcer healing rate.

Conventional doses of H₂-blockers cannot produce ulcer healing rates that are comparable with omeprazole over a four-week period, although eight weeks of treatment usually produces a 95% ulcer healing rate. However, even this does not produce the almost predictable healing result that is achieved by omeprazole.

Could the H₂-blockers ever produce results similar to those of omeprazole? The answer probably is 'yes'. If multiple doses of ranitidine are given each day, e.g. 300 mg q.d.s. (Lanzon-Miller et al, 1987b), then it is possible to produce a profound decrease of 24-hour intragastric acidity, very similar to that of omeprazole. An alternative approach to the problem might be to develop some form of delayed release preparation of ranitidine, so that the drug's rapid elimination from the body (its half-life in blood is only two hours) is no longer a problem.

Potential Benefits of Profound Inhibition of 24-hour Acidity

There are a number of clinical problems where the conventional doses of H₂-receptor blockers have failed to produce a clear clinical benefit. Perhaps the most common problem is *oesophagitis, oesophageal stricture and oesophageal ulceration*. Although the H₂-blockers can benefit some patients, the benefit is unpredictable (Gledhill and Hunt, 1987). Early experience with omeprazole has suggested that this agent may be almost as effective in this indication as in duodenal ulceration (Wetzel et al, 1986; Klinkenberg et al, 1987).

The same cannot be said of gastric ulceration—the H₂-blockers speed the healing of gastric ulceration, albeit rather more slowly than duodenal ulceration (Classen et al, 1985); early experiments with omeprazole for the management of benign gastric ulceration suggest that the results are very much like those achieved with conventional H₂-blockers (Colin-Jones, 1987)—perhaps acid is not quite such an important factor in the aetiology of gastric ulceration.

Profound inhibition of 24-hour acidity may also help patients with 'intractable duodenal ulceration' (Pounder, 1984). There is some evidence that omeprazole may benefit this type of patient (Tytgat et al, 1987). Omeprazole has a persisting action; in duodenal ulcer patients even a week after stopping the drug there is still a degree of inhibition of gastric acid secretion (Sharma et al, 1984a). Hence, a patient can probably have remarkably poor compliance, yet receive effective control of gastric acid secretion, week by week. It is possible that one of the reasons why omeprazole may be successful for 'resistant duodenal ulcers' is that the drug itself can tolerate relatively poor compliance.

Potential Disadvantages of Profound Inhibition of Gastric Acid Secretion

There are three types of potential disadvantage that may follow profound inhibition of gastric acid secretion. Firstly, the gastric barrier to enteric infection is broken; secondly, the stomach itself may get colonised by bacteria, with subsequent development of endogenous nitrosamines; thirdly, there is a reciprocal relationship between intragastric acidity and plasma gastrin concentration—as acidity falls so plasma gastrin rises. It is now clear that gastrin may act as a trophic hormone on the enterochromaffin-like (ECL) cells of the gastric mucosa, and that in pernicious anaemia the ECL hyperplasia may form discrete carcinoid tumours (Hodges et al, 1981; Morgan et al, 1983; Helling and Wood, 1983; Stockbrugger et al, 1983; Goldfarb et al, 1983; Caruso et al, 1984; Harvey et al, 1985; Lethola et al, 1985; Borch et al, 1985, 1986; Larsson et al, 1986a; Carney et al, 1983; Bordi et al, 1974, 1978; Sokcia et al, 1975).

Enteric infections

Clinical case reports can be used to demonstrate that a loss of gastric acidity leaves the small and large intestine liable to enteric infection. Examples of such infections include *Salmonella, Clostridium difficile, Clostridium botulinum* and giardiasis (Howden and Hunt, 1987). It is clear that intragastric acid has an important protective role and it normally sterilises the contents of the stomach. Hence, it would seem unwise for any patient to travel in areas where there is low food hygiene, whilst taking any agent that causes a profound 24-hour decrease in intragastric acidity. Indeed, the latest H_2-blocker regimens (Ireland et al, 1984; Lee et al, 1986; Ryan et al, 1986; Delattre et al, 1985; Capurso et al, 1984), using a pulse of profound inhibition during the night and early morning, together with normal acidity during the day, would seem absolutely ideal for such travellers—they would have plenty of acid about whilst they take each of the three main meals, yet they would have control of acid during the night, at a time when they should not be ingesting enteric pathogens!

Bacterial colonisation of the stomach

There is considerable literature concerning the development of bacterial colonisation of the stomach, following control of intragastric acidity (Milton-Thompson et al, 1982; Sharma et al, 1984b). It seems that bacteria can be found in the stomach almost immediately after acid is eliminated, but colonisation will only occur when there is unremitting control of acidity for many days or weeks. Such colonisation has been observed during treatment with omeprazole, with an associated rise in intragastric nitrite and nitrosamine content (Sharma et al, 1984b). However, all these abnormalities were cleared within days of stopping omeprazole, as acid secretion returned to the stomach with consequent sterilisation of the gastric contents. Patients with pernicious anaemia have no acid in their stomach for many years, and they certainly have colonisation of the gastric contents (Drasar et al, 1969). Pernicious anaemia is a risk factor for gastric adenocarcinoma, but only after many years (Mosbech and Vidbaek,

1950; Ruddell et al, 1978). In this context, transient profound pharmacological control of intragastric acidity can be considered only a small problem.

Gastric carcinoids

Finally, much of the recent excitement in the pharmacological control of gastric acid secretion centres around the development of ECL cell (the commonest endocrine cell of the fundic mucosa of the stomach) hyperplasia and gastric carcinoids (Hakanson and Sundler, 1986). The role of this cell in man is unknown. In two-year toxicology experiments in the rat, omeprazole was found to be associated with ECL cell hyperplasia or the development of gastric carcinoids (tumours composed of ECL cells) (Ekman et al, 1985). Extensive experiments now show that in the rat proliferation of ECL cells can be induced by hypergastrinaemia—caused either by very high dose treatment with ranitidine or omeprazole (Larsson et al, 1986b), or long-term treatment with parenteral pentagastrin (Blom, 1986).

We have recently completed experiments in 12 duodenal ulcer patients before and after treatment with 28 days of omeprazole 20 mg o.m. or ranitidine 150 mg b.d. (Lanzon-Miller et al, 1987a), which caused 24-hour integrated plasma gastrin concentration to rise from 328 pmol/h/l pretreatment to 799 and 1519 pmol/h/l on the 28th day of treatment, respectively. There was a significant inverse correlation between the 24-hour intragastric acidity and 24-hour plasma gastrin concentration—as acidity dropped, so there was a steady rise of plasma gastrin concentration.

Similar studies have also been carried out in eight pernicious anaemia patients (Lanzon-Miller et al, 1987a) eating identical meals and studied under the same environmental conditions; these patients had far higher gastrin concentrations than observed in either omeprazole- or ranitidine-treated patients—by comparison, the median value for the pernicious anaemia patients was 9934 pmol/h/l. Although these antisecretory drugs do produce a rise of plasma gastrin in man, this rise is of a completely different order to that observed in patients with pernicious anaemia.

Pernicious anaemia patients are relevant because, after many years of achlorhydria and hypergastrinaemia, they may develop either ECL cell hyperplasia or rare carcinoid tumour formation (Hodges et al, 1981; Morgan et al, 1983; Helling and Wood, 1983; Stockbrugger et al, 1983; Goldfarb et al, 1983; Caruso et al, 1984; Harvey et al, 1985; Lethola et al, 1985; Borch et al, 1985, 1986; Larsson et al, 1986a; Carney et al, 1983; Bordi et al, 1974, 1978; Sokcia et al, 1975). However, there is no clear report that any patient with hypergastrinaemia and pernicious anaemia has ever developed a carcinoid tumour that has caused fatal metastases. Hence, it appears that drug-induced hypergastrinaemia, using the conventional H_2-blockers or omeprazole, should not be a problem for the management of simple peptic ulceration.

Conclusions

The original regimen using cimetidine (200 mg t.d.s. with 400 mg at night) was devised as a technique to produce an economic profound decrease of 24-hour intragastric acidity. Over the following years there was a gradual evolution in management; the whole dose of either drug is now given at bedtime—ranitidine 300 mg or cimetidine 800 mg. However, both regimens only heal approximately 80% of duodenal ulcers after four weeks of treatment; there remain a number of clinical situations where conventional doses of H_2-blockade offer little benefit.

The development of omeprazole, a drug that can cause a sustained profound decrease of 24-hour acidity, has shown that higher ulcer healing rates can be achieved by profound pharmacological control of acid secretion. It has now been shown that, by giving more frequent and larger doses of ranitidine, a similar control of intragastric acidity can be achieved using a conventional drug.

The disadvantages of a profound decrease of intragastric acidity are the possibility of enteric infection following ingestion of contaminated food, the colonisation of the stomach by bacteria, and drug-induced hypergastrinaemia. Where there is the chance of clinical benefit none of these potential problems is sufficiently serious to withhold short-term, drug-induced profound inhibition of gastric acid secretion.

References

Bardram L, Thomsen P and Stadil F (1986) Gastric endocrine cells in omeprazole-treated and untreated patients with the Zollinger Ellison syndrome. *Digestion* **35** (suppl 1), 116–22.

Black JW, Duncan WAM, Durant CJ, Ganellin CR and Parsons ME (1972) Definition and antagonism of histamine H_2-receptors. *Nature* **236**, 385–90.

Blom H (1986) Effects of omeprazole on normal and regenerating gastric mucosa in the rat. A light and electron microscope study. *Scand. J. Gastroenterol.* **21** (suppl 118), 70–1.

Borch K, Renvall H and Liedberg G (1985) Gastric endocrine cell hyperplasia and carcinoid tumors in pernicious anaemia. *Gastroenterology* **88**, 638–48.

Borch K, Renvall H, Liedberg G and Andersen BN (1986) Relations between circulating gastrin and endocrine cell proliferation in the atrophic gastric fundic mucosa. *Scand. J. Gastroenterol.* **21**, 357–63.

Bordi C, Cocconi G, Toyni R, Vezzadini P and Missale G (1974) Gastrin endocrine proliferation. Association with the Zollinger-Ellison syndrome. *Arch. Pathol.* 274–9.

Bordi C, Gabrielli M and Missale G (1978) Pathological changes of endocrine cells in chronic atrophic gastritis. An ultrastructural study on peroral gastric biopsy specimens. *Arch. Pathol. Lab. Med.* **102**, 129–35.

Burland WL, Hawkins BW and Beresford J (1980) Cimetidine treatment for the prevention of recurrence of duodenal ulcer: an international collaborative study. *Postgrad. Med. J.* **56**, 173–6.

Capurso L et al (1984) Comparison of cimetidine 800 mg once daily and 400 mg twice daily in acute duodenal ulceration. *Br. Med. J.* **289**, 1418–20.

Carney JA, Go VLW, Fairbanks VF et al (1983) The syndrome of gastric argyrophil carcinoid tumours and non-antral gastric atrophy. *Ann. Intern. Med.* **99**, 761–6.

Caruso MP, Beardwood D, Maxwell R and Wagner C (1984) Gastric atrophy and carcinoid tumours. *Ann. Intern. Med.* **100**, 459.

Classen M, Dammann HG, Domschke W et al (1985) Omeprazole heals duodenal, but not gastric ulcers more rapidly than ranitidine. *Hepatogastro Enterology* **32**, 243–5.

Clissola SP and Campoli-Richards DM (1986) Omeprazole: a preliminary review of its pharmacodynamic and pharmacokinetic properties and therapeutic potential in peptic ulcer disease and Zollinger Ellison syndrome. *Drugs* **32**, 15–47.

Colin-Jones DG (1987) Medical treatment of peptic ulcer. In: Misiewicz JJ, Pounder RE and Venables CW (eds) *Diseases of the Gut & Pancreas*, Oxford: Blackwell, pp 288–315.

Cooperative Study (1984) Omeprazole in duodenal ulceration: acid inhibition, symptom relief, endoscopy healing, and recurrence. *Br. Med. J.* **289**, 525–8.

Delattre N et al (1985) Cimetidine 800 mg nocte in the treatment of acute duodenal ulceration. *Curr. Therap. M.* **37**, 677–84.

Drasar BS, Shiner M and McLeod GM (1969) Studies in the intestinal flora. *Gastroenterology* **56**, 71–9.

Duncan WAM and Parsons ME (1980) Reminiscences of the development of cimetidine. *Gastroenterology* **78**, 620–5.

Ekman L, Hansson E, Havu N et al (1985) Toxicological studies on omeprazole. In: Borg KO and Olbe L (eds) Omeprazole Book One. *Scand. J. Gastroenterol.* **20** (suppl 108), 53–69.

Gledhill T and Hunt RH (1987) Oesophagitis and hiatus hernia. In: Misiewicz JJ, Pounder RE and Venables CW (eds) *Diseases of the Gut & Pancreas*, Oxford: Blackwell, pp 137–53.

Gledhill T, Howard OM, Buck M, Paul A and Hunt RH (1983) Single nocturnal dose of an H_2-receptor antagonist for the treatment of duodenal ulcer. *Gut* **24**, 904–8.

Goldfarb JP, Gross F, Maxfield R, Rubin M and Janis R (1983) Gastric carcinoid: two unusual presentations. *Am. J. Gastroenterol.* **78**, 332–4.

Gustavsson S, Loof L, Adami HO, Myberg A and Nyren O (1983) Rapid healing of duodenal ulcers with omeprazole: double-blind dose-comparative study. *Lancet* **ii**, 124–5.

Hakanson R and Sundler F (1986) Mechanisms for the development of gastric carcinoids. *Digestion* **35** (suppl 1), 1–152.

Harvey RF, Bradshaw MJ, Davidson CM, Wilkinson SP and Davies PS (1985) Multifocal gastrin carcinoid tumours, achlorhydria, and hypergastrinaemia. *Lancet* **i**, 951–3.

Helling TS and Wood WG (1983) Gastric carcinoids and atrophic gastritis. Evidence for an association. *Arch. Surg.* **118**, 765–8.

Hodges JR, Isaacson P and Wright R (1981) Diffuse enterochromaffin-like (ECL) cell hyperplasia and multiple gastric carcinoids: a complication of pernicious anaemia. *Gut* **22**, 237–41.

Howden CW and Hunt RH (1987) Relationship between gastric secretion and infection. *Gut* **1**, 96–107.

Hunt RH, Howden CW, Jones DB, Burget DW and Kerr GD (1986) The correlation between acid suppression and duodenal ulcer healing. *Scand. J. Gastroenterol.* **21** (S125), 22–8.

Ireland A, Gear P, Colin-Jones DG et al (1984) Ranitidine 150 mg twice daily versus 300 mg nightly in treatment of duodenal ulcers. *Lancet* **ii**, 274–5.

Ivey KJ (1975) Anticholinergics: do they work in peptic ulcer? *Gastroenterology* **68**, 154–66.

Klinkenberg-Knol EC, Jansen JMB, Festen HPM, Meuwissen SGM and Lamers CBHW (1987) Double-blind multicentre comparison of omeprazole and ranitidine in the treatment of reflux oesphagitis. *Lancet* **i**, 349–51.

Lanzon-Miller S, Pounder RE, Hamilton MR et al (1987a) 24 hour intragastric acidity and plasma gastrin concentration before and during treatment with either ranitidine or omeprazole. *Aliment. Pharmacol. Therap.* **1**, in press.

Lanzon-Miller S, Pounder RE, Chronos NAF et al (1987b) Can high dose oral ranitidine eliminate intragastric acid, and what does it do to plasma gastrin? *Gastroenterology* **92**, in press (abstract).

Lanzon-Miller S, Pounder RE, Hamilton MR et al (1987c) 24 hour intragastric acidity and plasma gastrin concentration before and during treatment with either ranitidine or omeprazole. *Aliment. Pharmacol. Therapeut.* **1**, in press.

Larsson H, Carlsson E, Mattsson H et al (1986a) Plasma gastrin and gastrin enterochromaffinlike cell activation and proliferation. *Gastroenterology* **90**, 391–9.

Larsson H, Carlsson E, Mattsson H et al (1986b) Plasma gastrin and enterochromaffin cell activation and proliferation. *Gastroenterology* **90**, 391–9.

Lauritsen K, Rune SJ, Bytzer P et al (1985) Effect of omeprazole and cimetidine on duodenal ulcer. *N. Eng. J. Med.* **312**, 958–61.

Lee RI, Reed PI, Crowe JP et al (1986) Acute treatment of duodenal ulcer: a multicentre study to compare ranitidine 150 mg twice daily with ranitidine 300 mg once at night. *Gut* **27**, 1019–5.

Lehtola J, Karttunen T, Krekela I, Niemela S and Rasanen O (1985) Gastrin carcinoids with minimal or no macroscopic lesion in patients with pernicious anaemia. *Hepatogastroenterology* **32**, 72–6.

Milton-Thompson GJ, Ahmet Z, Lightfood NF et al (1982) Intragastric acidity, bacteria, nitrite and N-nitroso compounds before, during and after cimetidine treatment. *Lancet* **i**, 1091–5.

Morgan JE, Kaiser CW, Johnson W et al (1983) Gastric carcinoid (gastrinoma) associated with achlorhydria (pernicious anemia). *Cancer* **51**, 2332–40.

Mosbech J and Vidbaek A (1950) Mortality from and risk of gastric carcinoma among patients with pernicious anaemia. *Br. Med. J.* **2**, 390–4.

Multicentre Trial (1975) Treatment of duodenal ulcer by metiamide. *Lancet* **ii**, 779–81.

Pounder RE (1984) Duodenal ulcers that will not heal. *Gut* **25**, 697–9.

Pounder RE, Williams JG, Milton-Thompson GJ and Misiewicz JJ (1975a) Relief of duodenal ulcer symptoms by oral metiamide. *Br. Med. J.* **2**, 307–9.

Pounder RE, Williams JG, Milton-Thompson GJ and Misiewicz JJ (1975b) Twenty-four hour control of intragastric acidity by cimetidine in duodenal ulcer patients. *Lancet* **ii**, 1069–70.

Pounder RE, Williams JG, Milton-Thompson GJ and Misiewicz JJ (1976) Effect of cimetidine on 24-hour intragastric acidity in normal subjects. *Gut* **17**, 133–8.

Pritchard PJ, Yeomans ND, Mihaly GW et al (1983) Effect of daily oral omeprazole on 24 hour intragastric acidity. *Gastroenterology* **287**, 1378–9.

Ruddell WSJ, Bone ES, Hill MJ and Walters CL (1978) Pathogenesis of gastric cancer in pernicious anaemia. *Lancet* **i**, 521–3.

Ryan FP, Jorde R, Eshanulla RSB, Summers K and Wood JR (1986) A single night time dose of ranitidine in the acute treatment of gastric ulcer: a European multicentre trial. *Gut* **27**, 784–8.

Sharma BK, Walt RP, Pounder RE et al (1984a) Optimal dose of oral omeprazole for maximal 24 hour decrease of intragastric acidity. *Gut* **25**, 957–64.

Sharma BK, Santana IA, Wood EC et al (1984b) Intragastric bacterial activity and nitrosation before, during and after treatment with omeprazole. *Br. Med. J.* **289**, 717–9.

Sokcia E, Capella C, Vassallo G and Buffa R (1975) Endocrine cells of the gastric mucosa. *Int. Rev. Cytol.* **42**, 223–86.

Stockbrugger RW, Menon GG, Beilby JOW, Mason RR and Cotton PB (1983) Gastroscopic screening in 80 patients with pernicious anaemia. *Gut* **24**, 1141–7.

Tytgat GNJ, Lamers CBH, Hameeteman W, Jansen JMBJ and Wilson JA (1987) Omeprazole in ulcers resistant to histamine H$_2$-receptor antagonists. *Aliment. Pharmacol. Therap.* **1**, 31–8.

Walt RP, Male PJ, Rawlings J et al (1981) Comparison of the effects of ranitidine, cimetidine and placebo on the 24 hour intragastric acidity and nocturnal acid secretion in patients with duodenal ulcer. *Gut* **22**, 49–54.

Wetzel DJ, Dent J, Laurence BH et al (1986) Omeprazole heals oesophagitis: a placebo controlled trial. *Gut* **27**, A609.

Wyllie JH, Hesselbo T and Black JW (1972) Effects in man of histamine H$_2$-receptor blockade by burimamide. *Lancet* **ii**, 1117–20.

Key Developments in Gastroenterology
Edited by P. R. Salmon
© 1988 John Wiley & Sons Ltd

12

Recent Trends in Duodenal Ulcer

J. J. Misiewicz

The Middlesex Hospital, London

Plus ça change, plus c'est la même chose. The natural history and clinical attributes of duodenal ulcer diathesis may be changing. What has produced these changes we do not know, apart from attributing them to ill-defined environmental factors. Increased consumption of non-steroidal anti-inflammatory drugs (NSAIDs) has received much publicity, but their importance probably lies in increasing the incidence of complications of ulcers, not in causing them. Despite these highly interesting changes, acid secretion, as far as we know, apparently continues unchanged.

Duodenal ulcer remains a common disease and an important source of morbidity and mortality, especially in the elderly. The cause of the duodenal ulcer diathesis has continued to elude investigators, but several recent developments have provided additional information concerning the aetiology and the behaviour of the disease.

Secretion of Acid

Duodenal ulcers are strongly linked in the lay and also in many medical minds with acid secretion, or hyperacidity, whatever that may mean. Measurements of acid secretion continue to attract investigators in all parts of the world, but have not shed much light on the cause of duodenal ulceration. However, the old dictum of 'no acid, no ulcer' has stood the test of time and remains broadly true. It could well now be rephrased in a more stimulating way to read 'if acid, why ulcer?', because many patients with duodenal ulcer have acid outputs within the normal range. The various abnormalities of acid handling that have been documented in duodenal ulcer are summarised in Table 1, from which it will be apparent that in each category of abnormal acid response to a range of stimuli, only a proportion of subjects exhibit abnormal results; this proportion is highly variable. There are several reasons for this: the selection of patients and of the control subjects studied, as well as the nature of the stimuli used to promote the

Table 1

Variable of acid secretion	Number of studies	% range of subjects with abnormal response
MAO Pg or Hist. > normal	17	16–56
BAO > normal	7	10–38
Cephalic AO > normal	4	7–55
Low D50 to pentagastrin	6	0–45
Meal-stimulated AO normal	8	10–100

Modified from Lam (1984).

secretion of acid, must contribute to the variability of the data. Even after these are discounted, however, it is apparent that the demonstration of abnormal features of acid secretion in duodenal ulcer may be possible only in some patients. It is not known whether abnormally high secretion of acid to one stimulus predisposes to hypersecretion in response to other agonists, although it seems reasonable to assume that it does. The studies available in this field have been reviewed in detail by Lam (1984).

One of the problems of this area has been the technical difficulty of 24-hour measurements of acid *output*. This is in contrast to the relative ease with which 24-hour intragastric *acidity* can be recorded by intermittent gastric aspiration (Pounder et al, 1976), or by indwelling pH electrodes or telemetery (Merki et al, 1987). Feldman and Richardson (1986) studied patients with duodenal ulcer and normal controls and measured their basal, interprandial and nocturnal acid secretion by gastric aspiration, while meal-stimulated acid output was estimated using intragastric titration. At 408 ($\pm$62) mmol acid/24 h, the stomachs of the patients with duodenal ulcer secreted significantly more acid than the controls (208$\pm$19 mmol/24 h) and the significantly higher rate of acid secretion was

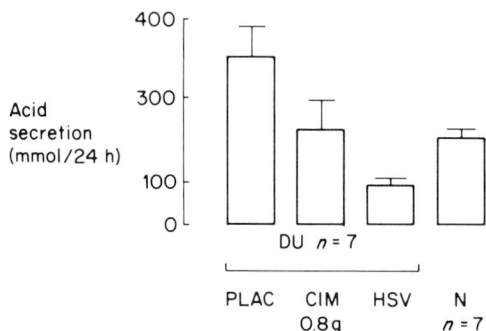

Figure 1. Twenty-four hour acid secretion in patients with duodenal ulcer and normals. PLAC = placebo; CIM = cimetidine; HSV = highly selective vagotomy. Reprinted with permission from Feldman and Richardson (1986) *Gastroenterology* **90**, 540–4. © The American Gastroenterological Association.

recorded during the day as well as during the night (Figure 1). Treatment with cimetidine decreased the 24-hour acid output significantly, but the 24-hour acid secretion was even lower in other subjects, who had had a parietal cell vagotomy. The results of this study are highly interesting, but have to be viewed in the light of the findings presented in Table 1. In other words, it would be unwise to extrapolate the concept of raised 24-hour acid output to all the patients with duodenal ulcer diathesis. For example, the percentage of patients with duodenal ulcer with maximal or peak acid output greater than the upper limit of normal following stimulation with histamine or pentagastrin varies from a low of 16–27% in studies done in the United States, to a high of 42–50% recorded in Scottish subjects (Lam et al, 1981).

Peak and maximal acid outputs are determined by the size of the parietal cell mass, which to some extent must also govern the magnitude of the 24-hour acid output, so although the measurements in the two sets of studies are not the same, they are related. Racial differences also must play a part: orientals with duodenal ulcer tend to have higher maximal acid outputs than westerners, even after correction of factors such as body weight, blood group, pyloric stenosis and family history (Lam et al, 1981). Such considerations serve to emphasise the concept that duodenal ulcer is a multifactorial disease. Unfortunately measurements of acid output are invasive, time consuming and labour intensive and this effectively prevents the prospective tailoring of treatment to a particular patient's level of acid secretion. In any case the results of treatment with acid-suppressing medication are so good that the need for such an exercise seems superfluous in all but the most resistant of duodenal ulcers. Moreover, a recent meta analysis of the published trials in duodenal ulcer seems to suggest that the most important factor determining the healing rate is the inhibition of nocturnal intragastric acidity (Jones et al, 1987).

The overriding importance of control of acid secretion in the practical management of duodenal ulcer disease is attested by the substantial decrease of acid output in patients with a successful parietal cell vagotomy, who have 24-hour acid secretion lower than those on the healing dose of cimetidine (Figure 1), and also by a study which shows that ulcers that did not heal after prolonged treatment with ranitidine or cimetidine healed after acid output was ablated with omeprazole (Tytgat et al, 1987). Most acid studies done recently deal with the effects of acid-suppressing medications and variations in drug administration schedules on 24-hour intragastric acidity, rather than address the pathophysiology of ulcer disease. However, such studies have been fundamental in providing objective data on which to base rational treatment dosages and timetables.

Pepsin and Mucus

Other major endogenous attack and defence factors affecting the integrity of the duodenal bulb mucosa have received further attention. Raised serum concentrations of pepsinogen-1 are significantly associated with duodenal ulcer, and concentrations of this substance above the upper limit of normal are present in more than 50% of patients (Samloff et al, 1975). Pepsinogen-1 has been shown to be immunochemically and electrophoretically heterogenous and divisible into two subclasses (alpha with two, and beta with one isozymogen); the genes coding for these variants have been proposed (Taggart and Samloff, 1987). Elevated serum pepsinogen-1 concentrations are associated with increased risk of duodenal ulcer, while raised concentrations of pepsinogen-2 and a low pepsinogen-1/pepsinogen-2 ratio are proposed as major risk factors for gastric ulcer (Samloff et al, 1986).

Gel filtration of human gastric mucus has shown a higher proportion of lower molecular weight mucous glycoprotein in samples from patients with gastric (and to a lesser extent also with duodenal) ulcer, suggesting a weaker gel structure, which is more liable to break down and less able to resist the passage of large molecules (Younan et al, 1982). Pearson et al (1986) studied degradation of mucus by pepsin and reported that pure human pepsin-1 (the peptic ulcer associated enzyme) digested gastric mucus glycoprotein faster than did pepsin-3, the principal human pepsin. Moreover, pepsin-1 still caused substantial mucolysis at pH 5.1, at which pepsin-3 was largely inactive. Gastric juice from patients with duodenal ulcer had mucolytic activity resembling that of pepsin-1, while activity of gastric secretion from controls resembled pepsin-3; gastric juice from duodenal ulcer patients decreased the viscosity of mucus more (Figure 2). These data suggest that gastric secretions from patients with duodenal ulcer attack the protective mucous gel more aggressively and are able to do this over a broader range of acidity than in healthy subjects. Although this study implies that raising the intragastric pH to around 5.0 would still leave pepsin-1 active in the ulcer patient, the apparent efficacy of low-dose antacid regimens in the

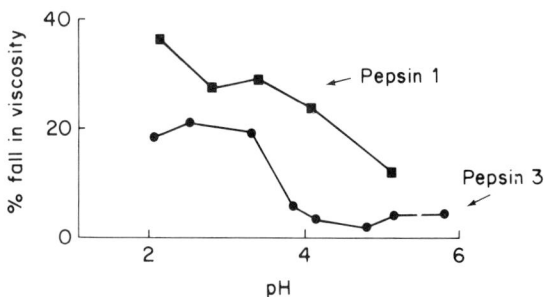

Figure 2. Differential activity of pepsin 1 and 3 over a pH range from 2 to 6. Mucus degradation is related to fall in viscosity. Pepsin-1 remains active above pH 4.
From Pearson et al (1986), with permission.

Lumen

Very
low pH   Soluble mucus

Near   Insoluble mucus-gel.
neutral   Permeable to small ions.
pH   Impermeable to pepsin
                                                                          (molecular weight 35000).

Gastric mucosa

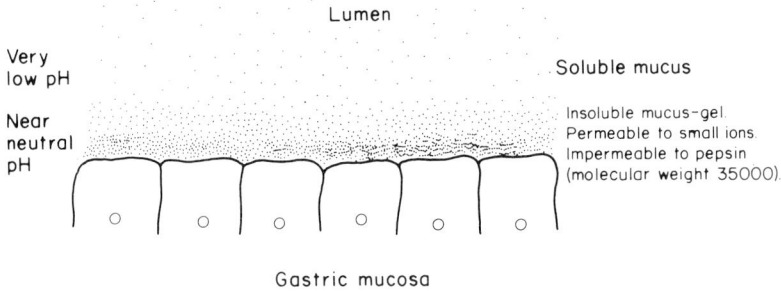

Figure 3. Mucus/bicarbonate components of the mucosal barrier. (See Hollander (1954), Heatley (1959), Allen and Garner (1982), and Rees and Turnberg (1982).)

healing and the prevention of relapse of duodenal ulcer must be borne in mind (Bardhan, 1986). However, the binding of pepsin by some antacids has not been quantified precisely. It has also to be remembered that the percentage of time at which intragastric pH is greater than 4 is low in patients with duodenal ulcer, although it may occur more frequently in gastric ulcer.

Bicarbonate

In addition to mucus, bicarbonate secreted by the pancreas and the duodenum may contribute to mucosal defence. The secretion of bicarbonate by the gastric and the duodenal mucosa may be an important component of the mucosal defence against acid. This may be so because the secreted bicarbonate does not diffuse freely into the gastric or duodenal lumen, but its luminalward spread is slowed down by the adherent layer of mucous gel. A steep pH gradient thus exists between the surface of epithelial cells and the lumen, with the pH at near neutrality at the mucosal surface, dropping steeply with each micron of distance away from the surface epithelium (Figure 3) (Hollander, 1954; Heatley, 1959; Allen and Garner, 1982; Rees and Turnberg, 1982). Isenberg et al (1987a) have recently shown that the human duodenum—studied with a multilumen tube perfusion system with occlusive balloons—secretes bicarbonate, the amount secreted being greater in the proximal duodenum. This work has now been extended (Isenberg et al, 1987b) to examine the effect of perfusing the duodenum with acid on the output of bicarbonate in subjects with and without duodenal ulcer; subjects with ulcers secrete less bicarbonate in their proximal duodenum in response to an acid stimulus (Figure 4). The basal output of bicarbonate of some 143 μmol/cm/h was increased by infusion of hydrochloric acid into the proximal or the distal duodenal perfusion segment. Bicarbonate output was also stimulated by intraluminal infusions of synthetic prostaglandin E1 (misoprostol).

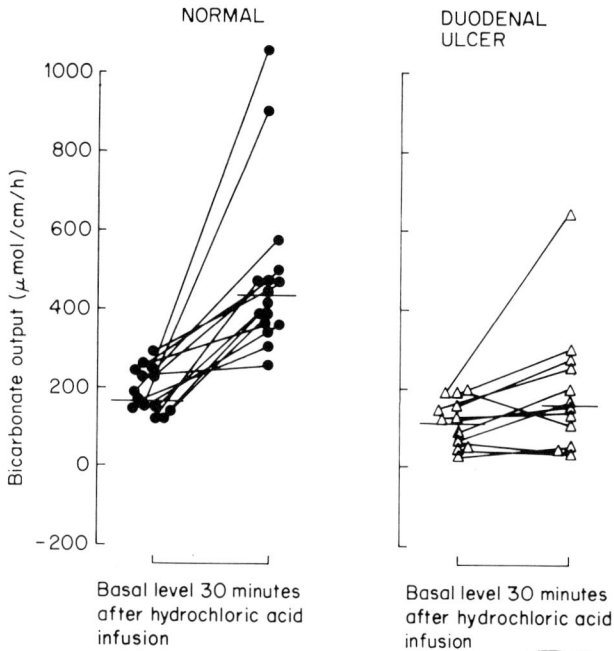

Figure 4. Secretion of bicarbonate by the proximal duodenum in response to acid perfusion. From Isenberg et al. Reprinted, by permission of the *New England Journal of Medicine* **316,** 374–8 (1987).

Campylobacter pylori

Although bicarbonate can be accepted as a factor contributing to mucosal defences, it somewhat paradoxically also provides an ecosphere in which *Campylobacter pylori* can flourish. This rather fastidious spiral flagellated organism has been recently rediscovered and has been the subject of intense research activity. *Campylobacter pylori* is found on the surface of gastric, but not of intestinal, epithelium and its presence is highly associated with antral gastritis and also with duodenal ulceration; it can be eradicated temporarily with bismuth, or with antibiotics, but its importance in ulcer causation, healing and relapse has not yet been settled (Axon, 1986; McNulty et al, 1986; O'Connor et al, 1986). The subject is dealt with in detail in Chapter 9.

Prostaglandins

Prostaglandins are present in the cells of the duodenal epithelium, but then they can be synthesised by any nucleated mammalian cell. NSAIDs suppress the synthesis of prostanoids by inhibiting the cyclooxygenase enzyme systems within the cells. Acute injury of the gastric mucosa by many noxious agents can be prevented by pretreatment with prostaglandins at doses that do not inhibit the secretion of acid. This cytoprotective property of exogenous prostaglandins has led to intense interest in their possible usefulness as therapeutic agents for duodenal ulcer. In general however, prostaglandin analogues have to be given in doses high enough to inhibit acid output before increased rates of ulcer healing can be shown in humans. Thus cytoprotection, or adaptive cytoprotection, may operate to prevent mucosal injury but does not seem to be active in the healing of a pre-existing ulcer crater (Hawkey and Walt, 1986). Measurements of prostanoid synthesis in human duodenal biopsy material is open to errors because of technical problems and the observations published so far have been conflicting, with some studies suggesting deficiencies in the mucosal content of some prostanoids (Hillier et al, 1985), while normal results have been obtained by others. It may be difficult to accept intrinsic prostanoid deficiency in subjects not deprived of dietary essential fatty acids. At present the role of prostaglandins in the causation of duodenal ulcer is not clear, but their deficiency may turn out to be important in an interesting area which concerns the rising incidence of perforation and acute gastrointestinal haemorrhage in people given NSAIDs.

Smoking and Anti-inflammatory Drugs

Smoking and the consumption of NSAIDs—two environmental factors which adversely affect the outcome of peptic ulceration—have been pinpointed recently. Smoking seems to decrease the rate of healing of duodenal ulcer in some, but not in all, clinical trials of standard ulcer treatment. Smokers also have more and earlier relapses of previously healed ulcers (Sontag et al, 1984). The mechanism of the deleterious effect of smoking on the outcome of duodenal ulcer is not known. The effects of cigarette smoking on the plasma concentrations of ranitidine and cimetidine are not very impressive (Boyd et al, 1987) and the effect of smoking on gastric acid secretion is, if present, very slight. How smoking affects defence factors, such as mucus and bicarbonate, is uncertain, nor is it established whether the effect of smoking could be mediated by changes in the mucosal circulation.

Analysis of the Hospital Inpatient Enquiry (HIPE) records has shown that between 1957 and 1977 admission and mortality rates for peptic ulcer had fallen in England and Wales (Coggon et al, 1981). Studies of these and similar variables performed more recently have shown changing, and to some extent worrying, features. Analysis of 230 people aged over 60 years admitted with bleeding peptic ulcers to hospitals in Nottingham (Somerville et al, 1986) has shown that non-aspirin NSAIDs were taken twice as often by the patients with bleeding than by community controls (relative risk 2.7; 95% confidence limits 1.7–4.4), or by hospital controls (relative risk 3.8; 95% confidence limits 2.2–6.4). Examination of the most recently available data shows that elderly people, and especially

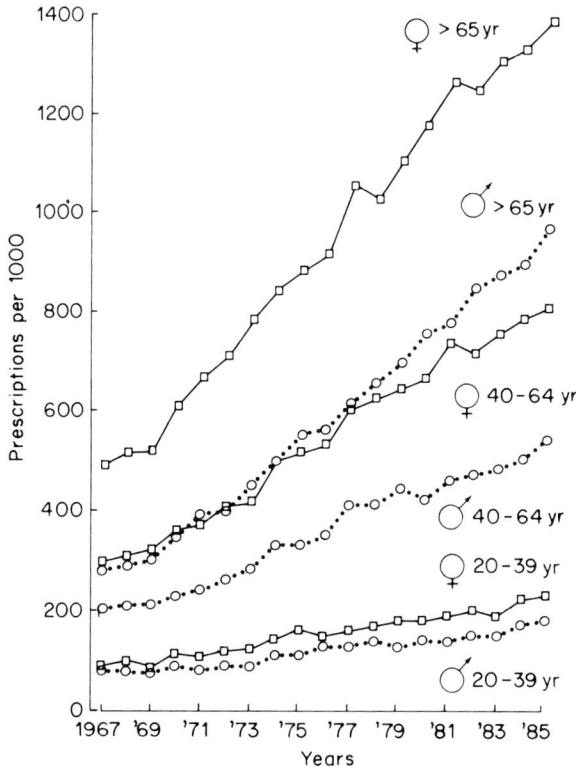

Figure 5. Age-specific NSAID prescription rates. From
Walt et al (1986), with permission.

women, are increasingly susceptible to perforation of peptic ulcer. Perforation
rates of duodenal ulcer have more than tripled in women aged 75 or over, and
have doubled in those aged 65 to 74 since 1958 (Watt et al, 1986). These observations are supported by another study, which confirms the association with
older age and the consumption of NSAIDs (Collier and Pain, 1985). Age-
specific prescription rates of NSAIDs shows a steep rise for the years 1967 to
1985, the number of prescriptions per 1000 increasing most in those aged 65 or
over, the highest rise being present in prescriptions given to women (Figure 5).
These adverse reactions must be balanced against the undoubted relief of the
symptoms of arthropathy produced by treatment with NSAIDs, and the still
relative rarity of serious unwanted effects, when considered in the context of the
total number of prescriptions issued; surveillance studies suggest that the
frequency of ulcer complications may be less than 1 per 10 000 prescriptions.
However, bleeding and perforated peptic ulcers carry a high mortality to which
the older population are particularly susceptible, while the number of

prescriptions for these agents is increasing. Now that the patients who are at high risk have been identified, prospective studies of prophylactic therapy are necessary. The problem there is that initial trials of standard anti-ulcer remedies in this area have so far been disappointing. Special care is needed when giving NSAIDs to older patients, especially to women and to those with a pre-existing peptic ulcer; these agents should not be prescribed for non-specific and ill-defined musculoskeletal syndromes in the high-risk groups. This is a counsel of perfection and not easy to follow in practice, as it is the older women who seem to need NSAIDs most often.

The points above emphasise that although the efficacy of treatment of duodenal ulcer has perceptibly advanced since the introduction of H_2 histamine receptor antagonists, there is no room for complacency. Several of the areas mentioned in this short review are discussed in more detail in Chaper 10.

References

Allen A and Garner A (1982) Gastric mucus and bicarbonate secretion and their possible role in mucosal protection. *Am. J. Physiol.* **242**, G183–348.

Axon ATR (1986) Campylobacter pyloridis: what role in gastritis and peptic ulcer? *Br. Med. J.* **293**, 772.

Bardhan KD (1986) Multicentre Study. Can antacids prevent duodenal ulcer relapse? *Gut* **27**, A612.

Boyd EJS, Johnston DA, Wormsley KG et al (1987) The effects of cigarette smoking on plasma concentrations of gastric antisecretory drugs. *Aliment. Pharmacol. Therap.* **1**, 57–65.

Coggon D, Lambert P and Langman MJS (1981) 20 years of hospital admissions for peptic ulcer in England and Wales. *Lancet* **i**, 1302–4.

Collier D St J and Pain JA (1985) Non-steroidal anti-inflammatory drugs and peptic ulcer perforation. *Gut* **26**, 359–63.

Feldman M and Richardson CT (1986) Total 24-hour gastric acid secretion in patients with duodenal ulcer. Comparison with normal subjects and effects of cimetidine and parietal cell vagotomy. *Gastroenterology* **90**, 540–4.

Hawkey CJ and Walt RP (1986) Prostaglandins for peptic ulcer: a promise unfulfilled. *Lancet* **ii**, 1084–6.

Heatley NG (1959) Mucosubstance as a barrier to diffusion. *Gastroenterology* **37**, 313–23.

Hillier K, Smith CL, Jewell R, Arthur MPJ and Ross G (1985) Duodenal mucosa synthesis of prostaglandins in duodenal ulcer disease. *Gut* **26**, 237–40.

Hollander F (1954) The two component mucus barrier. *Arch. Intern. Med.* **93** 107–20.

Isenberg JI, Hogan DL, Koss MA and Selling JA (1987a) Human duodenal mucosal bicarbonate secretion. Evidence for basal secretion and stimulation by hydrochloric acid and a synthetic prostaglandin E1 analogue. *Gastroenterology* **91**, 370–9.

Isenberg JI, Selling JA, Hogan DL and Koss MA (1987b) Impaired proximal duodenal mucosal bicarbonate secretion in patients with duodenal ulcer. *N. Engl. J. Med.* **316**, 374–8.

Jones BD, Howden CW, Burget DW, Kerr GD and Hunt RH (1987) Acid suppression in duodenal ulcer, a meta-analysis to define optimal dosing with antisecretory drugs. *Gut* **28** (in press).

Lam SK (1984) Pathogenesis and pathophysiology of duodenal ulcer. In Isenberg JI and Johansson C (eds) *Clinics in Gastroenterology*; Peptic ulcer. London: Saunders. Vol. 13, 447–72.

Lam SK, Hasan M, Sircus W et al (1981) Comparison of maximal acid output and gastrin response to meals in Chinese and Scottish normal and duodenal ulcer subjects. *Gut* **21**, 324–8.

McNulty CAM, Dear JC, Crump B et al (1986) Campylobacter pyloridis and associated gastritis: investigator-blind placebo-controlled trial of bismuth salicylate and erythromycin succinate. *Br. Med. J.* **293**, 645–9.

Merki H, Witzel L, Harpe K et al (1987) Single dose treatment with H_2 receptor antagonists: is bedtime administration too late? *Gut* **28**, 451–4.

O'Connor HJ, Dixon MF, Wyatt JI et al (1986) Effect of duodenal ulcer surgery and enterogastric reflux on campylobacter pyloridis. *Lancet* **ii**, 1178–81.

Pearson JP, Ward R, Allen A, Roberts NB and Taylor WH (1986) Mucus degradation by pepsin; comparison of mucolytic activity of human pepsin 1 and pepsin 2. *Gut* **27**, 243–9.

Pounder RE, Williams JG, Milton-Thompson GJ and Misiewicz JJ (1976) Effect of cimetidine on 24 hour intragastric acidity in normal subjects. *Gut* **17**, 133–8.

Rees WDW and Turnberg LA (1982) Mechanism of gastric mucosal protection: a role for the 'mucus-bicarbonate' barrier. *Clin. Sci.* **62**, 343–8.

Samloff IM, Liebmann WL and Donitch NM (1975) Serum group 1 pepsinogens by radioimmunoassay in control subjects and patients with peptic ulcer. *Gastroenterology* **69**, 83–90.

Samloff IM, Stemmermann GN, Heilburn LK et al (1986) Elevated serum pepsinogen I and II levels, differ as risk factors for duodenal and gastric ulcer. *Gastroenterology* **90**, 570–6.

Somerville K, Faulkner G and Langman M (1986) Non-steroidal anti-inflammatory drugs and bleeding peptic ulcer. *Lancet* **i**, 462–4.

Sontag S, Graham DY, Belsito A et al (1984) Cimetidine, cigarette smoking and recurrence of duodenal ulcer. *N. Engl. J. Med.* **31**, 689–95.

Taggart RT and Samloff IM (1987) Immunochemical, electrophoretic and genetic heterogeneity of pepsinogen 1. *Gastroenterology* **92**, 143–50.

Tytgat GNJ, Lamers CBHW, Hameeteman W et al (1987) Omeprazole in peptic ulcers resistant to histamine H_2-receptor antagonists. *Aliment. Pharmacol. Therap.* **1**, 31–8.

Walt R, Katschinski B, Logan R, Ashley J and Langman M (1986) Rising frequency of ulcer perforation in elderly patients in the United Kingdom. *Lancet* **i**, 489–92.

Younan F, Pearson J, Allen A and Venables C (1982) Changes in the structure of the mucus gel on the mucosal surface of the stomach in association with peptic ulcer disease. *Gastroenterology* **82**, 269–80.

Key Developments in Gastroenterology
Edited by P. R. Salmon
© 1988 John Wiley & Sons Ltd

13

Gastroduodenal Bicarbonate Secretion

C. J. Shorrock
W. D. W. Rees
Hope Hospital, University of Manchester School of Medicine, Salford

The surface mucosa of the healthy stomach and duodenum is continually being exposed to high concentrations of a corrosive mixture of hydrochloric acid, pepsin and, in many healthy subjects, transient reflux of bile which exposes the stomach to the detergent effect of bile salts. In the duodenum, acid emptying from the stomach is rapidly neutralised but still pH values of around 2 can occur in the proximal duodenum for variable lengths of time. These aggressive damaging luminal factors along with damaging ingested agents such as non-steroidal anti-inflammatory drugs (NSAIDS) and alcohol must be balanced by defensive and repair processes to maintain mucosal integrity (Figure 1). In peptic ulcer disease an increase in the damaging aggressive components acid and pepsin is found in only a minority of patients and these factors do not alter during or after spontaneous healing. This has focused attention on gastroduodenal defence mechanisms in an attempt to understand the aetiology and pathogenesis of this common condition.

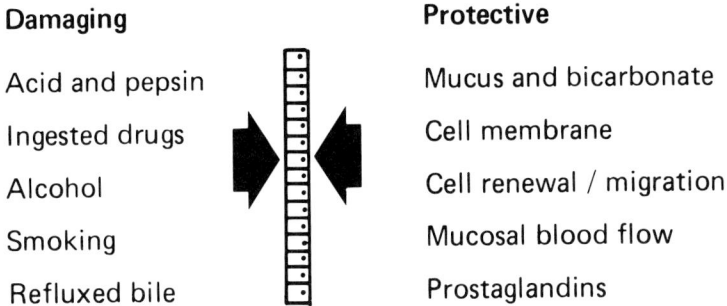

Damaging	Protective
Acid and pepsin	Mucus and bicarbonate
Ingested drugs	Cell membrane
Alcohol	Cell renewal / migration
Smoking	Mucosal blood flow
Refluxed bile	Prostaglandins

Figure 1. Damaging and protective factors that may operate in the human stomach.

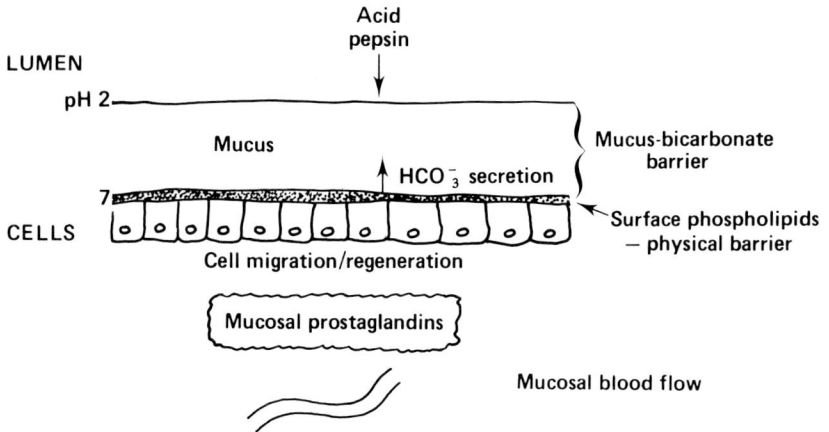

Figure 2. The possible components of gastroduodenal mucosal defence.

Gastroduodenal Defence Mechanisms

The concept of mucosal defence has come a long way since the work of Pavlov (1898) and Florey and co-workers (1939) who performed important experiments on the ability of the duodenum to resist acid and pepsin. A number of factors have now been identified as being important in mucosal resistance to acid and pepsin (Figure 2). The first line of defence is the thick layer of adherent mucus gel which covers gastric and duodenal mucosa. This was thought to contribute very little to overall gastroduodenal defence until the demonstration of alkali secretion by the underlying epithelial cells into the mucus layer (Flemstrom, 1977). This 'mucus-bicarbonate' barrier sustains a pH gradient between the lumen and cell surface such that epithelial cells are maintained at pH 7 to 8 despite intraluminal acid. The epithelial cells form a second line of defence and since the pH gradient may be overwhelmed by physiological concentrations of intraluminal acid, this mechanism may be important in maintaining mucosal integrity. The physical properties of the apical cell membrane and intercellular junctions (Davenport et al, 1964) and the presence of surface active phospholipids on the membrane may be responsible for preventing hydrogen ions from diffusing into the mucosa by providing a physical barrier to their movement. Furthermore, epithelial cells are capable of rapid turnover and migration and may breach a defect in the epithelium within a few hours.

The aftermath of mucosal damage may generate a further defence mechanism, a thick layer of mucus containing sloughed epithelial cells together with passive movement of bicarbonate-rich fluid from damaged mucosa. This may prevent exposure of undamaged cell nests to acid and thus aid re-epithelialisation. Finally, mucosal blood flow plays a vital role in maintaining epithelial integrity

(Guth, 1980) and studies have shown that increasing or decreasing mucosal blood flow will reduce or enhance susceptibility to damage respectively. Blood flow, in addition to delivering oxygen and essential nutrients to the cells, also supplies bicarbonate and may remove diffused hydrogen ions.

This ability of the gastric mucosa to protect itself from intraluminal contents has been termed 'cytoprotection' and there is evidence that the stomach may enhance this protection in response to mild damaging agents—'adaptive cytoprotection'. Although the precise physiological control mechanisms for mucosal protection have not been defined, there is evidence that local prostaglandin metabolism, especially prostaglandin E2, plays an important role (Miller, 1983). The release of neurotransmitters and hormones may also contribute to or modulate the defence mechanisms.

Historical Background

The existence of gastric bicarbonate secretion was suggested as early as 1892 by Schierbeck and in 1898 by Pavlov who suggested that 'alkaline mucus' lined gastric mucosa neutralising luminal acid. Because of the magnitude of this secretion it was dismissed as providing any significant contribution to mucosal defence. Little new work arose in this area until 1939 when Florey and co-workers demonstrated that the duodenum was much better at resisting instillation of gastric juice than distal small bowel. In the absence of pancreato-biliary secretion, this acid resistance of the duodenum was proposed as being due to neutralisation by bicarbonate secretion from Brunner glands or from the mucosa itself. The occurrence of gastric bicarbonate secretion was demonstrated by Grossman (1959) studying antral pouches, and by Hollander (1954) in fundic pouches after inhibition of H^+ secretion by vagotomy and antrectomy. In 1959, Heatley suggested that protection of the gastric epithelium from acid could be

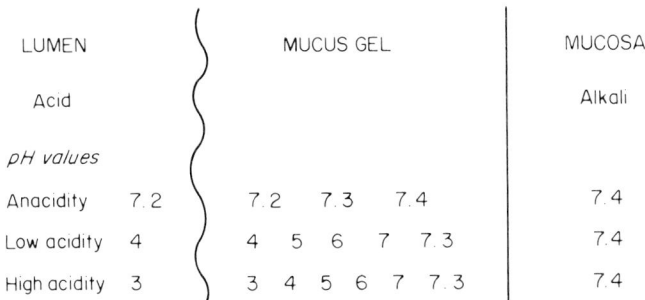

LUMEN		MUCUS GEL			MUCOSA
Acid					Alkali
pH values					
Anacidity	7.2	7.2	7.3	7.4	7.4
Low acidity	4	4	5	6	7	7.3	7.4
High acidity	3	3	4	5	6	7	7.3	7.4

Figure 3. The pH gradient across gastric mucus gel postulated by Heatley (1959).

afforded by bicarbonate secretion from mucosa into the mucus gel layer adherent to it. This would provide a zone of low turbulence supporting a pH gradient across it generated by acid–bicarbonate interaction (Figure 3). At this time a pH gradient could not be demonstrated experimentally and the hypothesis became superseded by the 'mucosal barrier' hypothesis of Code and Davenport (Davenport et al, 1964). They considered that a gastric mucosal barrier, formed by the apical membrane of surface cells together with the tight junctions linking adjacent cells, was responsible for the low permeability of the mucosa to ions.

A major problem in attempting to measure gastric bicarbonate secretion is the simultaneous but much greater secretion of hydrogen ions. It was not until the development of potent inhibitors of gastric acid secretion that it really became feasible to measure gastric bicarbonate secretion. The gastric juice of patients with achlorhydria (Gardham and Hobsley, 1970) as well as normal subjects (Kristensen, 1975) was known to contain bicarbonate, but pioneering work by Flemstrom (1977) proved the existence of bicarbonate secretion from fundic and antral mucosa by a metabolically dependent process as well as by passive diffusion. He used isolated pieces of frog gastric mucosa stripped of muscularis externa and mounted in Ussing chambers. These findings have subsequently been corroborated by other workers, and gastric bicarbonate secretion has now been documented in a large number of experimental models, including the intact human stomach (Flemstrom, 1981; Rees et al, 1982). More recently, bicarbonate secretion from proximal duodenal mucosa has been demonstrated both in vitro and in vivo (Flemstrom, 1980; Isenberg et al, 1986).

The Significance of Gastroduodenal Bicarbonate Secretion

The existence of alkali secretion by the stomach and proximal duodenum has now been established, but since its magnitude is so small compared with acid output its physiological significance remains in doubt. If secreted directly into the lumen, the bicarbonate would be overwhelmed by intraluminal acid and confer little protection on underlying epithelial cells. An unstirred layer which confines acid–bicarbonate interaction close to the cell surface is therefore essential and evidence has recently emerged that gastric mucus provides such a zone. Although Hollander (1954) and Heatley (1959) had postulated the existence of a mucus gel layer containing acid–bicarbonate interaction, proof of its existence was not forthcoming until the last five years. The elaborate studies of Allen provided better understanding of mucus structure and function, and in particular helped explain the visco-elastic properties of the gel. Subsequent studies clarified the structure of the gel and its interaction with small ions, such as hydrogen and sodium. Until recently there were no methods for measuring the mucus gel thickness in 'unfixed' preparations. Two methods have now been published which enable accurate quantitation of the unstirred layer covering the surface epithelium. The first of these used a slit lamp and pachymeter, which is

Table 1. Effects of mucus gel on the diffusion of hydrogen ions. The experiments used layers of pig mucus gel mounted in modified Ussing chambers (Williams and Turnberg, 1980).

	Thickness (cm)	D (moles/cm^2/s)
Saline	0.1	$6.2 \pm 0.3 \times 10^{-5}$
	0.2	$6.96 \pm 0.51 \times 10^{-5}$
Mucus	0.1	$1.75 \pm 0.34 \times 10^{-5}$
	0.2	$1.75 \pm 1.16 \times 10^{-5}$
	$p < 0.0001$	

normally used to measure corneal thickness, while the second employed phase contrast microscopy. Since the first method may also measure fluid covering the gel, recordings of gel thickness by this technique have been greater in magnitude than those by phase contrast microscopy, which detects the gel layer only. Despite these discrepancies, the methods have clearly documented the existence of a substantial layer of gel, some 5–10 times the height of epithelial cells, which covers the entire surface of the gastroduodenal mucosa. The mucus gel layer is a dynamic structure and is reduced by mucolytic agents and increased by prostaglandins (Kerss et al, 1982), stretching of the mucosa and the ulcer healing drug, carbenoxolone. Experiments on the interaction between mucus gel and small ions have shown that it does not simply act as an unstirred layer of water (Pfeiffer, 1981; Williams and Turnberg, 1980). The glycoprotein molecules appear to retard the movement of H^+, so that diffusion of such ions across the mucus gel is four times slower than through a similar layer of water (Table 1).

Mucus gel therefore provides an ideal zone for containing the acid–bicarbonate interaction close to the cell surface. Mucus gel and bicarbonate secretion clearly complement each other in that either alone would confer little mucosal protection. In combination, however, these components prevent direct exposure of the epithelial cells to luminal acid, and this has been confirmed experimentally using pH-sensitive microelectrodes advanced across mucus of gastric and duodenal mucosa. Such experiments have shown a marked pH gradient from lumen to cell surface in both the stomach and proximal duodenum (Williams and Turnberg, 1981; Takeuchi et al, 1983; Ross et al, 1981). The resulting protective zone produced by bicarbonate transport into mucus gel has been termed the 'mucus–bicarbonate' barrier.

Mechanisms of Gastric and Duodenal Bicarbonate Secretion

Gastric bicarbonate secretion

Bicarbonate is secreted by surface epithelial cells of the stomach at a basal rate of about 5–10% of maximum acid output (Flemstrom, 1981). Initial experimental

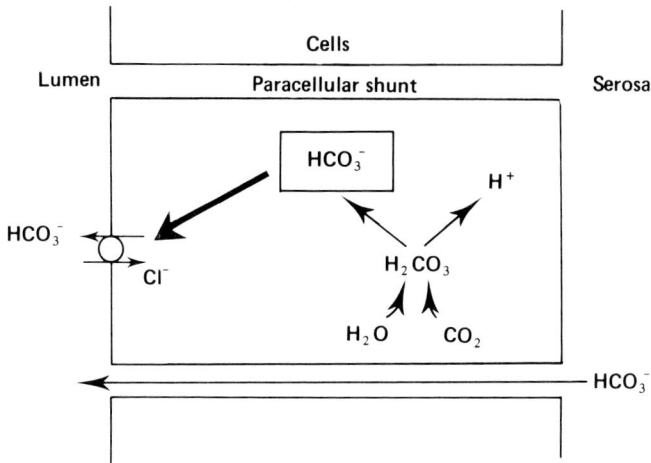

Figure 4. Transport mechanisms for bicarbonate across gastric epithelium.

work with isolated amphibian mucosa, and more recently with mammalian mucosa and in vivo preparations (Flemstrom et al, 1982a; Smeeton et al, 1983), has shown that bicarbonate ions are transported across gastric mucosa either by a metabolically dependent transcellular route, or through intercellular channels by passive diffusion (Figure 4). The gastric fundus appears to transport bicarbonate by a metabolically dependent process only, secretion being abolished or substantially decreased by anoxia or inhibitors of tissue metabolism (potassium cyanide and dinitrophenol) (Flemstrom, 1977). The antrum on the other hand transports about one-third of its bicarbonate by passive diffusion.

Transcellular transport of ions may occur by an electrogenic process, whereby transfer of ions across a membrane results in alteration of the potential difference and short circuit, or by an electroneutral process whereby an ion is exchanged for one of similar charge without altering mucosal potential difference. In vitro studies suggest that active bicarbonate secretion by fundus and antrum probably occurs by chloride–bicarbonate exchange at the apical membrane of surface epithelial cells (Flemstrom, 1982; Flemstrom et al, 1982b). Thus, cellular transport of bicarbonate by gastric mucosa may be inhibited by agents which interfere with this ion exchange process, such as SITS, DIDS and furosemide or by depleting luminal chloride ions. The bicarbonate necessary for this exchange is probably generated within the fundic cells by the action of carbonic anhydrase since it has been observed that bicarbonate secretion by intact mucosa and monolayers of surface epithelial cells are more sensitive to luminal than to serosal side administration of acetazolamide (Flemstrom, 1977; Rutten et al, 1983). In the antrum, however, there is also some evidence that extracellular bicarbonate may be an important source of transported bicarbonate.

Duodenal bicarbonate secretion

In the duodenum the situation appears more complex. It is possible that Brunner glands contribute to epithelial bicarbonate secretion although some of the characteristics originally attributed to Brunner gland alkaline secretion, such as inhibition by aspirin (Russel and Jones, 1974) or stimulation by VIP (Kirkegaard et al, 1981), have been demonstrated for duodenal mucosa devoid of these glands. Pancreatobiliary secretion also contributes to net luminal alkali. Isolated duodenal mucosa secretes alkali at about twice the rate of basal gastric alkali secretion (Flemstrom and Garner, 1982). As in the gastric antrum approximately 30–40% of basal secretion is due to passive diffusion across a transepithelial concentration gradient while most of the remaining basal secretion occurs by an electrogenic transport process (Simpson et al, 1981a, 1981b), unlike the chloride–bicarbonate exchange of gastric fundus and antrum (Figure 5). In the duodenum, endogenous production of bicarbonate by the surface cells contributes little to overall alkalinisation, in that acetazolamide in a dose causing 99% inhibition of carbonic anhydrase fails to inhibit basal duodenal bicarbonate secretion. In this tissue, extracellular bicarbonate appears to be the main source of transported alkali. Although basal bicarbonate secretion from proximal duodenal mucosa occurs by these two transport processes, there is evidence that a chloride–bicarbonate exchange mechanism may be activated by certain stimulants, such as the hormone GIP and endogenous opiates.

Control of Gastroduodenal Bicarbonate Secretion

The demonstration of an alkaline environment adjacent to surface epithelium in the stomach and duodenum and its dependence on mucosal bicarbonate

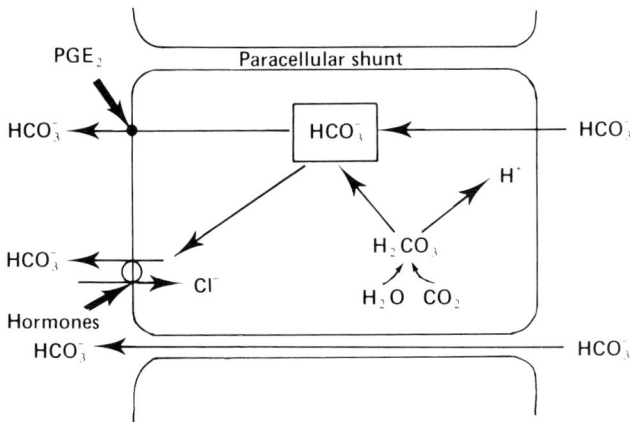

Figure 5. Transport mechanisms for bicarbonate across duodenal epithelium.

Table 2. Control of bicarbonate secretion.

	Gastric	Duodenal
Luminal factors:	Acid	Acid
	Bile	Distension
	Distension	
	Food	
Cellular factors:	cGMP	cAMP
	Calcium	Calcium
	Carbonic Anhydrase	
Neural factors:	Enteric neurones	Enteric neurones
	Vagus	Vagus
	Cholinergic	Sympathetic
		Enkephalinergic
Humoral factors:		
Local	Prostaglandins	Prostaglandins
		Endorphins
Systemic	CCK	Glucagon
	Glucagon	Neurotensin
	VIP	VIP

secretion has led to considerable interest in the mechanisms which regulate this secretion. There is a vast amount of information available on the neurohumoral regulation of gastric acid secretion but comparatively little data on the factors which modulate alkali secretion. Furthermore, the majority of this information has been derived from in vitro or in vivo studies where non-physiological amounts of neurotransmitters or hormones have been used to produce a secretory response. Studies on intact animals and the use of physiological stimuli are extremely limited and it is difficult to decide at present which of the neurohumoral agents studied play a role in regulating gastroduodenal bicarbonate secretion. Recent studies, however, suggest that vagal stimulation and luminal acid probably play an important role in controlling both gastric and duodenal bicarbonate secretion (Forsell et al, 1985; Isenberg et al, 1986). Gastric bicarbonate secretion may be stimulated by the cholinergic agonist carbachol (Flemstrom et al, 1984), and there is evidence that intracellular generation of cyclic GMP and extracellular calcium may also be important (Table 2). Sham feeding has been shown to increase gastric bicarbonate secretion (Forsell et al, 1985; Feldman, 1985) while electrical stimulation of the vagi enhances both gastric and duodenal alkalinisation (Nylander et al, 1985; Jonsson et al, 1985). These responses were inhibited by cholinergic antagonists, such as atropine and benzilonium bromide. Further evidence for the neural control of gastroduodenal bicarbonate secretion has been derived from studies where either electrical stimulation of the nucleus ambiguus or intrahypothalamic infusion of corticotrophin-releasing factor have been shown to significantly increase bicarbonate production by stomach or proximal duodenum (Pagani et al, 1984; Gunion et al, 1985). Our own studies suggest an important role for cholinergic neurones in regulating duodenal bicarbonate secretion. Using the technique of electrical field stimulation we have shown that activation of neurones in isolated duodenal mucosa significantly increases the rate of alkali secretion, a response which is prevented by atropine (Crampton et al, 1986a). Although at an early stage, these pieces of information do indicate that vagal cholinergic pathways not only affect gastric acid output but also enhance gastroduodenal bicarbonate production.

This raises the intriguing possibility that changes in acid output may be coupled with simultaneous changes in gastroduodenal alkali production. In addition to simultaneous neural stimulation of acid and alkali secretion there is evidence that other mucosal mechanisms may couple these secretory processes. Using a Heidenhain pouch model, Garner and Hurst (1981) showed that acidification of the gastric remnant resulted in stimulation of bicarbonate secretion by the pouch. Since the pouch was largely denervated their results suggest that acidification of gastric mucosa releases a humoral factor that increases bicarbonate production by the surface epithelium. This phenomenon has been termed 'autoregulation' and in subsequent laboratory studies, this was confirmed in vitro using two mucosal strips mounted in parallel in a modified Ussing chamber (Heylings, 1983, 1984). In these experiments there was clearly no neural connection between the mucosa, confirming release of a factor or factors from one mucosa which acted upon the second. Since the response could be reduced by adding indomethacin to the bathing solutions, it was suggested that prostaglandins generated by gastric mucosa exposed to acid were responsible for the alkaline response. The autoregulation of bicarbonate secretion by topical acid has since been demonstrated in both the human stomach and proximal duodenum in vivo (Isenberg et al, 1986; Crampton et al, 1986b). Although it has been suggested that liberation of mucosal prostaglandins may also be responsible for these observations, the evidence is as yet unconvincing and it is possible that, in the intact organ, neural mechanisms or other local factors play an important role.

Another possible link between acid and alkali secretion by gastric mucosa exists. It has been observed that gastric mucosa actively secreting acid is more resistant to damage than non-secreting mucosa. Thus exposure of gastric mucosa to histamine stimulates acid production and also increases the resistance of the mucosa to damage by intraluminal acid. This response is blocked by H_2 antagonists and it has been suggested that the resistance to damage is produced by the 'alkaline tide' liberated by secreting parietal cells. Release of bicarbonate from parietal cells would in theory provide more interstitial bicarbonate for transport by the surface epithelium. Furthermore, parenteral infusion of bicarbonate has also been shown to protect gastric mucosa from damage (Kivilaakso, 1981). The possibility thus exists that the secretory activity of parietal cells is coupled with the secretory activity of surface epithelial cells by changes in interstitial bicarbonate delivery. Clearly, further studies are necessary to substantiate such a theory.

The importance of other neurohumoral factors in regulating gastroduodenal bicarbonate secretion remains uncertain. The gastrointestinal hormones CCK, pancreatic glucagon and GIP influence gastric alkalinisation while in the duodenum VIP and GIP, but not secretin, have been shown to stimulate output. Noradrenaline and isoprenaline also modify gastroduodenal alkali secretion and these responses have been incriminated in the pathogenesis of stress ulceration. However, as yet, the physiological or pathological significance of these preliminary experimental observations remains uncertain. The stomach and duodenum have been shown to contain enkephalin-like immunoreactivity in both mucosal endocrine cells and neurones. Recently, two groups of investigators have shown stimulation of duodenal bicarbonate secretion by opioids and the possibility exists that endogenous opiates also regulate duodenal alkalinisation (Rees et al, 1986; Flemstrom et al, 1986).

It is obvious from the above discussion that the control of gastroduodenal bicarbonate secretion is poorly understood and it seems inevitable that investigators will need to follow the 'painstaking' trail of physiologists and clinicians who helped clarify the regulatory mechanisms for acid secretion.

Prostaglandins and Gastroduodenal Bicarbonate Secretion

Exogenous prostaglandins have been shown to protect gastric mucosa from the effects of a variety of damaging agents (Robert, 1979) and the local generation of these substances within gastric mucosa has been considered responsible for mucosal adaptation to attack by mild irritants (adaptive cytoprotection) (Robert, 1980). The protective effects of prostaglandins, and more recently other therapeutic agents, on gastroduodenal mucosa has been termed 'cytoprotection'. Although such an application of the word is technically incorrect, its use in this context has now become widespread and 'cytoprotective' appears to be the 'in phrase' for describing anti-ulcer drugs which do not influence acid secretion.

It has been suggested that one mode of action of prostaglandins is to enhance the 'mucus–bicarbonate' barrier and there is evidence that both the mucus gel and bicarbonate secretion components are influenced by these agents (Bickel and Kaufman, 1981; Smeeton et al, 1983). In early experiments exogenous prostaglandins (E2 and F2α) were shown to stimulate basal bicarbonate secretion and prevent its inhibition by NSAIDs using isolated amphibian mucosa. Furthermore, the inhibition of bicarbonate secretion produced by NSAIDs was attributed to a decrease in endogenous prostaglandin synthesis by gastroduodenal mucosa. These observations have, largely, been subsequently confirmed using mammalian mucosa and in the intact human stomach. As previously discussed there is also evidence linking autoregulation of gastroduodenal alkali secretion by topical acid with endogenous prostaglandin synthesis. Since recent studies have shown that a number of currently used ulcer healing drugs (aluminium containing antacids, colloidal bismuth and sucralfate) are capable of enhancing both gastroduodenal prostaglandin synthesis and bicarbonate secretion, there is mounting evidence linking endogenous prostaglandin, gastroduodenal bicarbonate secretion and mucosal protection.

More detailed analysis of the information, however, reveals a number of important flaws in the hypothesis. Firstly, a number of prostaglandins protect gastroduodenal mucosa without influencing bicarbonate secretion. Secondly, careful microscopic evaluation of the protective effect of exogenous prostaglandins against damage by various topical agents suggests that the surface epithelium is not protected and that the major impact of such prostaglandins is submucosal. This would suggest that under such circumstances, prostaglandin-mediated effects on the 'mucus–bicarbonate' barrier contribute little to overall mucosal protection. This is particularly relevant for ethanol-induced mucosal damage. Finally, although certain ulcer-healing drugs may produce simultaneous increases in prostaglandin formation and bicarbonate secretion by gastroduodenal mucosa, there is conflicting evidence that these two processes are causally linked.

There is no doubt that certain exogenous prostaglandins increase both mucus gel thickness (Bickel and Kaufman, 1981) and bicarbonate secretion, leading to an enhanced pH gradient overlying gastric and duodenal epithelium (Flemstrom and Kivilaa, 1983). The importance of endogenous prostaglandin metabolism in the physiological control of bicarbonate secretion remains uncertain, and as yet there is insufficient evidence to link prostaglandin induced mucosal protection with enhancement of the 'mucus–bicarbonate' barrier. It has been established that prostaglandins influence a number of other protective mechanisms, such as surface active phospholipids (Hills et al, 1983) and mucosal blood flow (Guth, 1984), and different protective mechanisms may be called into action to deal with different damaging agents or even different concentrations of the same agent. Thus prostaglandin-induced enhancement of the 'mucus–bicarbonate' barrier may be important in protecting against acid and NSAIDs (depending on local concentrations) but of little significance in preventing damage by ethanol.

Clinical Significance of the Mucus–Bicarbonate Barrier

Although there is evidence that mucosal damage by bile salts and NSAIDs may, in part, be mediated by the adverse effects of these agents on the 'mucus–bicarbonate' barrier (Rees et al, 1981, 1983, 1984), there is very little information to link defects in the barrier with peptic ulcer pathogenesis.

The mucus gel structure in gastric ulcer patients has been demonstrated to be abnormal in that it contains less 'native' glycoprotein (Younan et al, 1982) while certain pepsins, which are more prevalent in duodenal ulcer disease, are capable of more aggressive digestion of the glycoprotein matrix (Pearson et al, 1986). In duodenal ulcer, the bicarbonate response to an acid load is defective (Isenberg et al, 1985) and an abnormal pH gradient in response to luminal acid has also been demonstrated in peptic ulcer patients indicating a deficit in the ability of these patients to maintain juxtamucosal neutrality in the face of luminal acidity (Quigley and Turnberg, 1987). Although this evidence points to a link between abnormalities of the mucus–bicarbonate barrier and ulcer pathogenesis, there is as yet no direct evidence for such a causal relationship.

The action of ulcer healing agents, which do not influence acid secretion, has also been linked to effects on gastroduodenal bicarbonate secretion. Prostaglandin analogues have recently been introduced as anti-ulcer drugs and, as previously discussed, have been shown to stimulate gastric and duodenal alkalinisation under certain experimental conditions. It is therefore conceivable that their therapeutic action depends in part on enhancement of the mucus–bicarbonate barrier. There is, however, evidence that some of the other currently available anti-ulcer drugs may heal ulcers by influencing the mucus–bicarbonate barrier. The antacid aluminium has been shown to produce marked stimulation of gastroduodenal alkali secretion in isolated mucosae. This observation is quite intriguing as it implies that in addition to providing an exogenous source of alkali to neutralise luminal acid, aluminium-containing antacids may also enhance the delivery of endogenous alkali into the mucus gel layer. Sucralfate and colloidal bismuth have also been shown to have similar effects, and since sucralfate contains aluminium it is tempting to speculate that a common denominator to these agents is a metallic cation. How these agents enhance alkali secretion remains uncertain, although there is evidence that they increase gastroduodenal prostaglandin synthesis and this in turn may activate bicarbonate transport.

If the mucus–bicarbonate barrier can be shown to play a role in the pathogenesis and healing of peptic ulcer disease then in future, the pharmaceutical industry may focus its attention on providing stimulants of bicarbonate, mucus or both as specific anti-ulcer drugs which would not significantly alter the luminal environment.

Other Factors Involved in Gastroduodenal Mucosal Defence

Surface epithelial cells

Epithelial cells play an important role in the first line defence of the stomach by the delivery of mucus gel and transport of bicarbonate. However, there is evidence that the epithelial cells have intrinsic barrier properties. Early studies by Davenport and Code in the 1960s suggested that the apical membrane and 'tight junctions' between epithelial cells were relatively impermeable to H^+ ions and therefore formed a barrier to diffusion. Some evidence suggests that fixed charges are present in channels within surface epithelium which impede the movement of positively charged ions such as H^+. More recent studies have documented the existence of surface active phospholipids providing the surface epithelium with a hydrophobic lining (Hills et al, 1983). This lining allows molecules of high lipid solubility to pass freely into the mucosa but retards the passage of water soluble ions such as H^+. Agents such as NSAIDs and bile salts increase mucosal permeability to H^+ ions and virtually eliminate surface hydrophobicity and these effects may be important in mediating their damaging action.

Mucosal repair (Lacy and Ito, 1984; Svanes et al, 1982)

The ability of surface epithelial cells to rapidly migrate across denuded lamina from cells in the gastric pits appears to be an important part of the mucosal defence system. After extensive destruction of superficial epithelial cells, experiments have shown complete re-epithelialisation within an hour. The repair process is protected from the damaging luminal environment by the overlying layer of mucus gel (Wallace, 1986) containing sloughed epithelial cells, and passive diffusion of bicarbonate. The mechanisms for regulating this re-epithelialisation process as yet remain unknown.

Blood flow (Guth, 1984)

Mucosal blood flow, by delivering oxygen, nutrients and bicarbonate to the surface epithelium and removing H^+ ions which have penetrated the mucus–bicarbonate and epithelial barriers, plays a vital role in protecting the gastric mucosa. There is considerable evidence that reduction in blood flow is important in mediating mucosal damage and duodenal mucosa appears more susceptible to reduction in blood flow than gastric mucosa. Prostaglandins can reduce or prevent the changes in gastric microcirculation produced by damaging agents and thus may be important in regulating mucosal blood flow. It is conceivable that regional variations in gastroduodenal mucosal blood flow is primarily responsible for the localised nature of peptic ulcer disease. Changes in the luminal environment and other defence mechanisms may therefore overwhelm these 'weak' areas of the mucosa while producing less marked damage elsewhere. Such a hypothesis, however, remains unproven.

Acknowledgements

The authors are grateful to the Department of Medical Illustration, Hope Hospital, for providing the figures. Dr Shorrock is a British Society of Gastroenterology Research Fellow.

References

Allen A (1981) Structure and function of gastric mucus. In Johnson LR, Christensen J, Grossman MI et al (eds) *Physiology of the Gastrointestinal Tract*, pp 617–39. New York: Raven Press.

Bickel M and Kaufman G (1981) Gastric mucus gel thickness: effect of distension, 16, 16-dimethylprostaglandin E2 and carbenoxolone. *Gastroenterology* **80**, 770–5.

Crampton JR, Gibbons LC and Rees WDW (1986a) Evidence for cholinergic modulation of duodenal bicarbonate secretion. *Gut* **27**(10), A1254.

Crampton JR, Gibbons LC and Rees WDW (1986b) Effect of acid on bicarbonate secretion by stomach in man: evidence for an autoregulatory reflex. *Gut* **27**(5), A592.

Davenport HW, Warner HA and Code CF (1964) Functional significance of gastric mucosal barrier to sodium. *Gastroenterology* **47**, 142–52.

Feldman M (1985) Gastric H$^+$ and bicarbonate secretion in response to sham feeding in humans. *Am. J. Physiol.* **248**, G188–91.

Flemstrom G (1977) Active alkalisation by amphibian gastric fundic mucosa in vitro. *Am. J. Physiol.* **233**, E1–12.

Flemstrom G (1980) Stimulation of HCO$_3^-$ transport in isolated proximal bull frog duodenum by prostaglandins. *Am. J. Physiol.* **239** (Gastrointest Liver Physiol 2), G198–203.

Flemstrom G (1981) Gastric secretion of bicarbonate. In: Johnson RL, Christensen J, Grossman MI, Jacobson ED and Schultz SD (eds) *Physiology of the GI tract*, vol 1, pp 603–14. New York: Raven Press.

Flemstrom G (1982) Properties of hormone and prostaglandin stimulated duodenal HCO$_3$ transport. In: Case MR, Garner A, Turnberg LA and Young JA (eds) *Electrolyte and Water Transport Across Gastrointestinal Epithelia*, pp 85–94. New York: Raven Press.

Flemstrom G and Garner A (1982) Gastroduodenal HCO$_3^-$ transport: characteristics and proposed role in acidity regulation and mucosal protection. *Am. J. Physiol.* **242** (Gastrointest Liver Physiol 5), G183–193.

Flemstrom G and Kivilaakso E (1983) Demonstration of a pH gradient at the luminal surface of rat duodenum in vivo and its dependence on mucosal alkaline secretion. *Gastroenterology* **84**, 787–94.

Flemstrom G, Garner A, Nylander O, Hurst BC and Heylings JR (1982a) Surface epithelial HCO$_3^-$ transport in vitro: effects of hormones and local transmitters. *Am. J. Physiol.* **243** (Gastrointest Liver Physiol 6), G348–58.

Flemstrom G, Heylings JR and Garner A (1982b) Gastric and duodenal bicarbonate transport in vitro: effects of hormones and local transmitters. *Am. J. Physiol.* **242** (Gastrointest Liver Physiol 5), G100–10.

Flemstrom G, Nylander O and Jedsted FG (1984) VIP and carbachol stimulates bicarbonate secretion by the surface epithelium in the rat duodenum in vivo (abst). *Acta Physiol. Scand.* **120**, 11a.

Flemstrom G, Jedstedt G and Nylander O (1986) ß-endorphin and enkephalins stimulate duodenal mucosal alkaline secretion in the rat in vivo. *Gastroenterology* **90**(2), 368–72.

Florey HW, Jennings MA, Jennings DA and O'Connor C (1939) The reactions of the intestine of the pig to gastric juice. *J. Path. Bact.* **49**, 105–23.

Forsell H, Stenquist B and Olbe L (1985) Vagal stimulation of human gastric bicarbonate secretion. *Gastroenterology* **89**, 581–6.

Gardham JR and Hobsley M (1970) The electrolytes of human alkaline human gastric juice. *Clin. Sci.* **39**, 77–87.

Garner A and Hurst BC (1981) Alkaline secretion by the canine heidenhain pouch in response to endogenous acid, some gastrointestinal hormones and prostaglandins. In: Gati T, Szollar LG and Ungvary CTY (eds) *Advances in Physiological Science*, vol 12. Nutrition, Digestion and Metabolism, pp 215–19. Oxford: Pergamon.

Grossman MI (1959) The secretion of the pyloric glands of the dog. Abstracts of the 21st International Congress of Physiological Sciences Buenos Aires. 1959, 226-8.

Gunion MN, Tache Y and Kauffman GL (1985) Intrahypothalamic corticotrophin-releasing factor (CRF) increases gastric bicarbonate content (abstr). *Gastroenterology* **88**, 1407.

Guth PH (1980) Gastric mucosal blood flow and resistance to injury. In: Holtermuller KH and Malagelada JR (eds) *Advances in Ulcer Disease*, pp 101-9. Amsterdam: Excerpta Medica.

Guth PH (1984) Local metabolism and circulation in mucosal defence. In: Allen A, Flemstrom G, Garner A, Silen W and Turnberg LA (eds) *Mechanisms of Mucosal Protection in the Upper Gastrointestinal Tract.* New York: Raven Press.

Heatley NG (1959) Mucosubstance and a barrier to diffusion. *Gastroenterology* **37**, 313-7.

Heylings JR (1983) A technique for studying the influence of luminal acid on frog gastric and duodenal bicarbonate transport in vitro. *J. Physiol.* **342**, 4-5.

Heylings JR, Garner A and Flemstrom G (1984) Regulation of gastroduodenal bicarbonate transport by luminal acid in the frog in vitro. *Am. J. Physiol.* **246** (Gastrointest Liver Physiol 9), G235-42.

Hills BA, Butler BD and Lichtenberger LM (1983) Gastric mucosal barrier: hydrophobic lining to the lumen of the stomach. *Am. J. Physiol.* **244** (Gastrointest Liver Physiol 7), G561-8.

Hollander HF (1954) The two-component mucus barrier. *Arch. Int. Med.* **94**, 107-20.

Hollander D, Tarnawski A, Gergeley H and Zipser RD (1984) Sucralfate protection of the gastric mucosa against ethanol induced injury—a prostaglandin mediated process. *Scand. J. Gastroent.* **19** (suppl. 10), 97-102.

Isenberg JI, Hogan DL, Selling JA and Koss MA (1985) Duodenal bicarbonate secretion in normal subjects and duodenal ulcer patients. *Dig. Dis. Sci.* **30**, A-17.

Isenberg JI, Hogan DI, Koss MA and Selling JA (1986) Human duodenal mucosal bicarbonate secretion. Evidence for basal secretion and stimulation by hydrochloric acid and a synthetic prostaglandin E1 analogue. *Gastroenterology* **91**, 370-8.

Jonsson C, Fandriks L, Nylander O and Flemstrom G (1985) Vagal stimulation of duodenal bicarbonate secretion in the rat in vivo (abst). *Acta Physiol. Scand.* **124** (suppl. 542), 360.

Kerss S, Allen A and Garner A (1982) A simple method for measuring thickness of the mucus gel layer adherent to rat, frog and human gastric mucosa: influence of feeding, prostaglandins, N-acetyl cysteine and other agents. *Clin. Sci.* **63**, 187-95.

Kirkegaard P, Lundberg JM, Poulsen SS et al (1981) Vasoactive intestinal polypeptidergic nerves and Brunner's gland secretion in the rat. *Gastroenterology* **81**, 872-8.

Kivilaakso E (1981) High plasma bicarbonate protects gastric mucosa against acute ulceration in the rat. *Gastroenterology* **81**, 921-27.

Kristensen M (1975) Titration curves for gastric secretion. *Scand. J. Gastroent.* **10** (suppl. 32), 1-149.

Lacy ER and Ito S (1984) Ethanol-induced insult to the superficial rat gastric epithelium: a study of damage and rapid repair. In: Allen A, Flemstrom G, Garner A, Silen W and Turnberg LA (eds) *Mechanisms of Mucosal Protection in the Upper Gastrointestinal Tract.* pp 49-55. New York: Raven Press.

Leung FW, Robert A and Guth P (1985) Gastric mucosal blood flow in rats after administration of 16, 16 dimethylprostaglandin E2 at a cytoprotective dose. *Gastroenterology* **88**, 1948-53.

Lichtenberger LM, Richards JE and Hills BA (1985) Effect of 16, 16 dimethylprostaglandin E2 on surface hydrophobicity of aspirin treated canine gastric mucosa. *Gastroenterology* **88**, 308-314.

Miller TA (1983) Protective effects of prostaglandins against gastric mucosal damage; current knowledge and proposed mechanisms. *Am. J. Physiol.* **245** (Gastrointest Liver Physiol 8), G601–23.

Nylander O, Fandriks L, Delbro D and Flemstrom G (1985) Effects of vagal stimulation on gastroduodenal bicarbonate secretion in the cat (abst). *Acta Physiol. Scand.* **123**, 30A.

Pagani FD, Norman WP, Kasbekar DK and Gillis RA (1984) Effects of stimulation of nucleus ambiguus complex on gastroduodenal function. *Am. J. Physiol.* **246**, G253–62.

Pavlov JP (1898) Die Arbeit der Verdauungdrusen Weisbaden: Bergman JF. Verlag.

Pearson JP, Ward R, Allen A et al (1986) Mucus degradation by pepsin comparison of mucolytic activity of human pepsin 1 and pepsin 3: implication in peptic ulceration. *Gut* **27**, 243–8.

Pfeiffer CJ (1981) Experimental analysis of hydrogen ion diffusion in gastrointestinal mucus glycoprotein. *Am. J. Physiol.* **240** (Gastrointest Liver Physiol 3), G176–82.

Quigley EMM and Turnberg LA (1987) The pH of the microclimate living human gastric and duodenal mucosa in vivo: Studies in control subjects and in duodenal ulcer patients. *Gastroenterology* (in press).

Rees WDW, Garner A, Vivian KHB and Turnberg LA (1981) Effect of sodium taurocholate on secretion by amphibian gastric mucosa in vitro. *Am. J. Physiol.* **240** (Gastrointest Liver Physiol 3), G245–9.

Rees WDW, Botham D and Turnberg LA (1982) A demonstration of bicarbonate production by the normal human stomach in vivo. *Dig. Dis. Sci.* **27**(11), 961–6.

Rees WDW, Gibbons LC and Turnberg LA (1983) Effects of NSAIDs and prostaglandins on alkali secretion by rabbit gastric fundus in vitro. *Gut* **24**, 784–9.

Rees WDW, Gibbons LC, Warhurst G and Turnberg LA (1984) Studies of bicarbonate secretion in the normal human stomach in vivo: effect of aspirin, sodium taurocholate and prostaglandin E2. In: Allen A, Flemstrom G, Garner A, Silen W, Turnberg LA (eds) *Mechanisms of Mucosal Protection in the Upper Gastrointestinal Tract.* New York: Raven Press.

Rees WDW, Gibbons LC and Turnberg LA (1986) Influence of opiates on alkali secretion by amphibian gastric and duodenal mucosa in vitro. *Gastroenterology* **90** (2), 323–7.

Robert A (1979) Cytoprotection by prostaglandins. *Gastroenterology* **77**, 761.

Robert A (1980) Prostaglandins and digestive diseases. In: Samuelson B, Rammwell P, Paoletti R (eds) *Advances in Prostaglandins and Thromboxane Research*, vol 8. New York: Raven Press. pp 1533–1541.

Ross IN, Bahari HMM and Turnberg LA (1981) The pH gradient across mucus adherent to rat fundic mucosa in vivo and the effects of possible damaging agents. *Gastroenterology* **81**, 713–8.

Russel TR and Jones RS (1974) The effect of aspirin on duodenal secretion. *Proc. Soc. Exp. Biol. Med.* **145**, 967–9.

Rutten MJ, Ito S, Rattner D and Silen W (1983) Transport by cultured monolayers of gastric surface epithelial cells. *Physiology* **26**, A-116 abstract).

Sanders MJ, Ayalon A, Roll M and Soll A (1985) The apical surface of canine chief cell monolayer resists H^+ back-diffusion. *Nature* **313**, 52–4.

Schierbeck NP (1892) Ueber Kohlemsaure im Ventrikel. *Scand. Arch. Physiol.* **8**, 437–4.

Simpson JNL, Merhav A and Silen W (1981a) Alkaline secretion by amphibian duodenum. I. General Characteristics. *Am. J. Physiol.* **240** (Gastrointest Liver Physiol 3), G401–8.

Simpson JNL, Merhav A and Silen W (1981b) Alkaline secretion by amphibian duodenum. II. Short circuit current and Na^+ and Cl^- fluxes. *Am. J. Physiol.* **240** (Gastrointest Liver Physiol 3), G472–9.

Smeeton L, Hurst B, Allen A and Garner A (1983) Gastric and duodenal HCO_3 transport in vivo: influence of prostaglandins. *Am. J. Physiol.* **245** (Gastrointest Liver Physiol 8), G751-9.

Svanes K, Ito S, Takeuchi K and Silen W (1982) Restitution of the surface epithelium of in vitro frog mucosa after damage with hyperosmolar sodium chloride. *Gastroenterology* **82**, 1409-26.

Takeuchi K, Magee D, Critchlow J et al (1983) Studies of the pH gradient and thickness of frog gastric mucus gel. *Gastroenterology* **84**, 331-40.

Venables CW (1986) Mucus, pepsin, and peptic ulcers. *Gut* **27**, 233-8.

Wallace JL and Whittle BJR (1986) Role of mucus in the repair of gastric epithelial damage in the rat. *Gastroenterology* **91**, 603-11.

Williams SE and Turnberg LA (1980) Retardation of acid diffusion by pig gastric mucus; a potential role in mucosal protection. *Gastroenterology* **79**, 299-304.

Williams SE and Turnberg LA (1981) Studies of the 'protective' properties of gastric mucus; evidence for a 'mucus–bicarbonate' barrier. *Gut* **22**, 94-6.

Younan F, Pearson J, Allen A and Venables C (1982) Changes in the structure of the mucus gel on the mucosal surface of the stomach in association with peptic ulcer disease. *Gastroenterology* **82**, 827-31.

Index

acetaldehyde 49, 50
acetazolamide 177
acquired immune deficiency syndrome (AIDS) 75, 77
  candidiasis, oral/oesophageal 78-9
  cholangitis 84, 85 (fig.)
  cytomegalovirus infections 81-3
    acute abdominal syndrome 83
    disseminated 83
  gastrointestinal conditions 80 (table)
  herpes virus infection 81-3
  liver conditions 80 (table)
  perianal ulcers 83
  perioral ulcers 83
  risk groups 75
  treatment 90-3
    bacterial infections 91
    fungal infection 92
    Kaposi's sarcoma 90
    protozoal infection 91
    viral infection 91, 92-3
  see also human immunodeficiency virus
ACTH 73
acyclovir 4, 91
  plus alpha interferon 7
adaptive cytoprotection 173
adenine arabinoside 4
adenine arabinoside monophosphate 4, 5 (fig.)
alcohol
  bottle of spirits content 47
  consumption, incidence of hepatic cirrhosis associated 47
  drug metabolism affected by 48
  hepatitis B enhancement 48
  liver damage see alcoholic liver disease
  paracetamol toxicity enhanced 63-4
  primary liver cancer associated 48
  'safe' daily consumption 47

alcoholic foamy degeneration (foamy fat syndrome) 62
alcoholic hepatitis 55-7
  acute virus hepatitis confused with 56
  clinical features 56
  histology 55-6
  laboratory tests 56-7
  see also alcoholic liver disease
alcohlic hyaline 50
alcoholic liver disease 47-66
  biochemical tests 51
  damage mechanisms 48-50
    acetaldehyde 49, 50
    alcoholic hyaline 50
    alcoholic metabolites 48-9
    hypermetabolic state 49-50
    immunological 50
    intracellular redox potential 49
    nutrition 50
  Dissë space collagenisation 52
  early recognition 50
  genetic susceptibility 48
  haematological changes 51
  hepatitis B associated 63
  liver biopsy 52
  portal hypertension associated 52
  screening questionaire, self-administered 50
  treatment 60-1
    early 60
    established liver disease 60-1
  vitamin A hepatic level 57
  women 47
  see also alcoholic hepatitis; fatty liver; hepatic cirrhosis
alcoholic patient, minimum daily food/vitamin requirements 59 (table)
alcoholism, occupational risk 47
alkaline phosphatase, serum 51

189